P9-DIG-779

WHAT WE DIDN'T EXPECT

What We Didn't Expect

Personal Stories About
Premature Birth

EDITED BY

Melody Schreiber

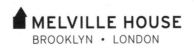

MELVILLE HOUSE
BROOKLYN · LONDON

What We Didn't Expect
First published in 2020 by Melville House Publishing

Copyright © Melville House, 2020
Copyright for individual essays belong to their respective authors
All rights reserved.

A version of "You're So Lucky" by Suzanne Kamata
appeared in *CALYX*.
A version of "New Year's Blessing" by Shawn Spruce
appeared in *Cherokee One Feather*.

First Melville House Printing: November 2020

Melville House Publishing
46 John Street
Brooklyn, NY 11201

and

Melville House UK
Suite 2000, 16/18 Woodford Road
London E7 0HA

mhpbooks.com
@melvillehouse

ISBN: 978-1-61219-860-6
ISBN: 978-1-61219-861-3 (eBook)

Library of Congress Control Number: 2020944450

Printed in the United States of America
Designed by Euan Monaghan

1 3 5 7 9 10 8 6 4 2

A catalog record for this book is available
from the Library of Congress

*For everyone we have met and
missed along the way.*

The beauty of life is in the unexpected.

Contents

Introduction

A few days after my tiny son first came home from the hospital, my exhausted brain finally remembered the books. Yes, the books! They would tell me what to do! I cracked open *What to Expect the First Year*—and immediately I started bawling.

My very premature baby faced a range of complications. His heart was failing, making him take about twice as many breaths as normal. Breastfeeding exerted him too much; instead, he was fed through a tube threaded through his nose. Often, his milk meals came right back up again when pressure from his swollen heart pushed against his stomach; I was terrified of leaving him alone for even a moment in case he choked on his vomit again. He was taking a host of potentially dangerous medications, and our lives revolved around appointments with specialists and his upcoming open-heart surgery. His diaper bag was packed with medical records—hospital transfer and discharge papers, notes on medications and side effects, instructions on feeding and following up with specialists.

None of this was what we had expected.

When my water broke at twenty-seven weeks and four days, everything changed. The drive to the hospital was nothing like I had anticipated for the past seven months—my belly was not enormous, I was not wracked by contractions. My husband drove nervously, cautiously, as fast as he could. The car was eerily silent. I kept my fingers spread over my stomach. *Not yet,* I told the son within. *Hold on just a little longer. Please, baby.*

After checking into the hospital, I settled into strict bed rest and began consulting with neonatologists about their plans for our baby's care once he arrived. There was so much we were learning on the fly; so much we never thought we'd need to know, now filling our heads and our hearts. Although we hoped he would wait—every day in utero was comparable to three days of growth and development in the neonatal intensive care unit (NICU), we learned—we knew the baby would not be full-term; if by some miracle the pregnancy reached thirty-four weeks, when his lungs and brain and body would be nearly mature, I would be induced in order to avoid infection and other complications. It was unnerving to know ahead of time he was going to be premature, while at the same time knowing there was nothing we could do to make his entry into the world any safer or less complicated. All we could really do was hope that he would wait. *Just a little longer.*

And he did; unlike the majority of pregnancies in which the water breaks early—a condition known as preterm premature rupture of membranes—my baby waited a full eighteen days. He was born twenty-nine weeks and six days into the pregnancy, and he was immediately taken to the NICU, where he would stay for more than two months.

There was nothing in the usual parenting books about how to address needs like his. On the contrary, those baby books were a painful reminder of the sharp turn our path had taken, and how far from the "normal" milestones we were drifting. For the first time in my life, books had failed me. I struggled to find stories that resonated with me—stories that would show me and my husband and our families a path forward in such a harrowing time. I felt intensely alone. Books had abandoned me, so I abandoned them; I put them back on the shelf, spines uncreased and pages smooth. It was another way in which this whole experience wouldn't go the way we had planned. We would simply have to go it alone.

But, I soon discovered, we were far from alone. Support and encouragement poured in from all around the country and the world; friends and family visited the hospital and our home as often as they could. Many people had no idea what to say or do in the face of premature birth and all of the complications that surrounded it, but that was okay; simply having them there, or reading their messages of love, helped more than we could ever tell them.

But there were others who reached out to say that they had some experience with preemies—a cousin or sibling or they themselves were born too soon. I had not realized how deeply prematurity had touched so many people's lives. Statistically, it made sense; one in ten babies are born early in the United States, so many people experience it in some way. Gradually, I patched together a network of friends who had been through this before, people I could message in a panic at ten in the evening or commiserate with at four in the morning. And I joined online groups with names like Preemie Friends and NICU Moms, learning terms like "tubie baby" and "heart warrior" and hearing even more heartbreaking and inspiring stories. These disparate voices helped us more than medical explanations; each distinctive viewpoint reassured us that we weren't the first to go through this—that there was light at the end of the tunnel.

Of course, the medical explanations were still important. I read the relevant portions of medical books on premature birth. I learned about chronic lung disease and developmental delays, about complications and fatality rates, about the alphabet soup of conditions and complications—RSV, RDS, IVH, PDAs (which are *not* public displays of affection, it turns out). But as a rule, I stayed as far away from these books as possible, only looking up certain terms and conditions—because the more I read, the more panicked I became about all of the many ways my little baby was vulnerable in this world. Far from providing relief or a sense of normalcy, these books usually only brought more fear. They were atlases of everything that could go wrong, compendia of potential catastrophes. I knew there were a few memoirs out there about babies born even smaller than my son, but I couldn't bear to read a whole book. What if that baby had needs nothing like my son's? What if something went wrong with the baby in the book—or what if she was fine, and it was my son who was unlucky? I was worried I would commit to a book and feel even worse as the baby's health yo-yoed, and also ... what new parents had time to read a whole book, anyway?

I dreamed of a collection that spoke to our situation—a book I could dip in and out of, flipping to the most resonant and applicable stories for us, a sort of Choose Your Own Adventure for navigating the NICU and beyond. I wanted to put our network of preemie voices into book form so other parents would not have to search as long as we did to find their people—to hear of others like them and how they dealt with the many challenges of early birth. Instead of turning to an atlas of fear, I wanted to provide a road map for getting through this and into the good part—the part when your baby smiles at you for the first time; the first day of freedom from the feeding tube or oxygen supplementation; the doctor's visit where they finally land on the growth chart; even the day when your grief over tremendous, unimaginable loss feels just a little bit less overwhelming.

/

Ten percent of babies are born prematurely in the United States—that's 400,000 families who go through this every year. But that one word, "preemie," encompasses a range of medical and cultural experiences. Even the terms used to describe prematurity are not set in stone, varying from hospital to hospital. In general, however, "micropreemie" usually describes babies born before twenty-six weeks, and "extremely premature" is used before twenty-eight weeks. A birth is usually considered premature before thirty-six weeks, but it is full-term between thirty-nine and forty weeks, leaving some strange gaps. Between thirty-six and thirty-seven weeks, a baby is "late preterm," and between thirty-seven and thirty-nine, "early term." All of these categories can get pretty confusing, and that's just the start of it.

Gestational age, or the number of weeks at which a baby is born, is important because it often plays an outsized role in how newborns fare. The earlier babies are born, the more challenges they face, from surviving the first few weeks to longer-term illnesses and diagnoses. However, medical advances in the past few decades have ensured that many, many more preemies than ever before survive and thrive.

There are also racial disparities before, during, and after pregnancy. For example, Black parents give birth prematurely 50 percent more than white parents in the United States. Each year, 13.6 percent of African American births happen early, compared with 9.0 percent of white births. Hispanic and Indigenous parents give birth early at higher rates as well—9.4 and 11.3 percent of the time, respectively.* The reasons for this are complex, but the accumulated stress of racism inflicts great harm on mental and physical health, and the discrimination frequently extends to medical treatment. Furthermore, research has shown, babies of color immediately begin facing racial discrimination in NICUs across the country.

The essays in this book reflect some of the diverse circumstances and experiences around premature birth. The contributors speak to the importance of recognizing and supporting good mental health, including postpartum anxiety, depression, and trauma; the significance of faith and community; making weighty choices with limited information; approaching loss and grief; and strengthening relationships with partners, friends, family, and health workers. Throughout the collection, they offer practical advice on raising a premature baby, navigating adoption, recognizing developmental delays, managing health insurance and financial decisions, and moving from guilt and blame to realizing that no one knows your child better than you do. No book can tell every story, but I hope this is the starting

---

* March of Dimes 2019 Report Card. Accessed at https://www. marchofdimes.org/mission/reportcard.aspx.

point for sharing how prematurity affects all of us—and how we can help preemie families (and their loved ones) navigate the difficult but also amazing time of welcoming a new child early.

These essays speak not just to premature children and their parents, but also to grandparents, aunts and uncles, cousins, and friends looking for answers and trying to find others' stories. They also provide another way for medical staff—doctors, nurses, specialists—to understand what families are going through and how best to communicate with and support them. (After all, it's not just the parents who deal with premature birth.) It is a reassuring chorus of the voices of preemies, family members, friends, and medical practitioners themselves.

What I wanted most after having a preemie was to be seen—to have our struggle to survive recognized, to feel a little less alone, to see our experiences reflected wherever I could find them. My hope is that the diverse and wide-ranging stories here will help those 400,000 other families through one of the most difficult—and beautiful—times in their lives.

Melody Schreiber
Washington, D.C.
November 2020

WHAT WE DIDN'T EXPECT

Miracle Baby

BY BECKY CHARNIAK

"The Greeks had no single term to express what we mean by the word 'life.' They used two terms that, although traceable to a common etymological root, are semantically and morphologically distinct: zoē, which expressed the simple fact of living common to all living beings (animals, men, or gods), and bios, which indicated the form or way of living proper to an individual or a group."

—Giorgio Agamben, Introduction, *Homo Sacer*

Looking back, I sometimes wonder why that morning took me by surprise. I was twenty-one weeks and four days into my pregnancy, and the path to that point had been so problematic already. There were sonogram images of our imperfectly shaped embryo, my excessive and hemorrhage-like bleeding, and the weeks of bed rest. I thought the icing on the cake was the night I passed a clot half the size of my fist while celebrating my birthday; we fished it out of the toilet and brought it to the doctor to confirm that our baby girl was not nestled inside. She somehow survived each scare without complication, and for a few weeks, my body had settled into normalcy. My obstetrician gave me the nod to start acting like this baby was going to be part of our future, so I got up the courage to make a nursery wish list.

On the day that we had planned to go to Babies "R" Us, I woke up and felt a rush of fluid come out of my body. I searched for clues: the color was clear, and the odor was not discernable. I tried desperately to convince myself that I had peed in my bed. All sorts of strange things happen that you don't know about in your first pregnancy, right? This was one of those rare moments when the hush and mystery surrounding the female body would work to my advantage, right? As I called my obstetrician, heard her tone, and passed more fluid in the bathroom, my head knew better. My water had broken.

It would take some time for my heart to catch up.

I walked back into the bedroom, my heart racing. I spread my hands wide and placed them on the bed alongside the soaked sheets. I leaned over and bent my head low. Quietly, but audibly, I said, "If You are out there, I need You now."

"Please," I begged, "If You are really there, if You can hear me, I need You now."

From a person who was raised Catholic, these words bordered on blasphemy. We learn at an early age that we shalt not put the Lord, our God, to the test. But that was exactly what I was doing. I may have said it politely, but "prove it" is what I meant. To this day, I cannot muster true remorse for that moment. I am not sorry because it was my deepest experience of human desperation, born from the strongest love I had ever known. If there ever was a time when I needed divine mercy, that was it.

It wouldn't be the first time I've shamelessly failed to tow the dogmatic line. I am what I have come to think of as a "Conflicted Catholic." Friends of mine sometimes refer to people like me as "Cafeteria Catholics," picking and choosing the elements of the faith that they find most appealing. But I expect I'm not the only believer for whom it is quite a bit more complicated than that. I don't break the rules because they are difficult to follow or because I am too proud to be guided by spiritual authority figures. Instead, I think the Roman Catholic Church fails in several practical, moral ways. As an analytical thinker and a social liberal, I see the Church as a fallible, powerful institution that can and does act in ways that conflict with Christ's message of love and service. I often revisit the passage from Romans 8 that I read at my grandfather's funeral: nothing can keep us from the love of God. The Church is no exception.

At the same time, the Catholic Church is the only spiritual home I have known. I value the vast amount of good works performed by its members; some of the most compassionate, selfless people I know are devout Catholics. I also have a deep veneration for the Sacraments and a connection with the Eucharist that cannot be matched in any other faith tradition. I can't just become a Unitarian and call it a day, even though sometimes that might be easier. I try my best to sort through the spiritual and logical conundrums. Always, I feel that my faith should be less about being right and more about becoming a better, more giving person.

Nearly an hour after waking on that cold January morning, I was admitted to the Catholic-affiliated hospital where my obstetrician happened to perform deliveries. An administrator, who showed no sense of urgency or interest, checked me in with all the standard paperwork. My husband provided my information while I stood in the doorway and cried. In an antepartum room, my obstetrician confirmed our fears. My water had broken, labor was imminent, and at this gestational age, our baby could not survive. An ultrasound machine was wheeled in, and there she was—our little girl, barely visible without the amniotic fluid to provide contrast. Her heart was beating normally, but my body could no longer give her what she needed. I had failed her.

One of the hospital workers arrived and told us that we would be offered a plot in their cemetery. I was both horrified and grateful. A few minutes later, she returned to ask me how far along I was in my pregnancy. She frowned when I answered, explaining that she was so sorry, but we were past the threshold for the hospital to make that bereavement offer to us. My dark sense of humor almost caused me to laugh at this: I had held onto my baby too long to earn her a free burial space but not long enough to live. At the same time, I understood. The land at the hospital's disposal was finite, and while they wanted to honor failed pregnancies, they had to draw a line somewhere.

The boundaries of the world we inhabit don't always leave room for living our ideals perfectly. Choices must be made.

The irony of belief knocking heads with reality was highlighted yet again when my doctor explained that one of my options was to be transported to a nearby hospital where they would be able to induce labor. This was a smart course of action because I had become susceptible to infection the moment my membrane ruptured. The concern was that I would develop sepsis, possibly damaging my uterus in a way that would make future pregnancies impossible. Or, worse, I could die. Since this was a Catholic hospital, they would not intervene unless the mother's life was in danger; the life living inside her was not expendable otherwise. With good reason, the doctors don't wait for a woman to be on the brink of death while knowing the baby can't survive outside of her anyway, and they offer the transfer to another hospital.

It was hard for me to take any of this seriously. All I really knew was that my baby was about to die, even while her heartbeat thundered along, strong inside of me. They were so certain that it was going to happen any minute. It would take everything in me just to exist, just not to dissipate into nothingness during this imminent moment of delivering my baby to death. The process was already set in motion. I didn't have it in me to speed it along. Unless I was actually starting to show signs of infection, I was incapable of choosing to induce labor. I stayed at the Catholic hospital. As long as our baby could hold on, I would too.

Left alone to process and grieve, I told my husband that she needed a name.

"It's Zoey, right?" I said.

"Yes," he said. It had been his favorite girl name ever since reading Salinger's *Franny and Zooey* in high school. I had liked it with a modified spelling well enough, but in that moment, it took on a new meaning for me. I recalled my days of studying political theory in graduate school, discussing Giorgio

Agamben's take on *zoē* as the natural state of living. Meaningful and beautiful on its own, as the life of a butterfly or an oak, but still less than a life that truly belongs to the human community of law and language. A body only, whose existence in and exclusion to a liminal, marginal space empowers and defines what it means to be an actualized participant in our political world.

Our baby was an asterisk. In the history of the human world, in the timeline of existence, she would be no more than a death certificate for the record books. Eleven days too old to qualify for a sympathy cemetery plot, and ten days too young to have any chance at survival. Yet for me, this speechless body with the beating heart, this face I may not gaze upon long enough to remember, would never exist at the margins. She had become the center of me. My life would revolve around her forever, even if it revolved around her absence. She was our everything, our Zoey.

/

In the two days that followed, I remained in the hospital. Our families came to be with us, playing card games and having conversations. It was a good distraction for my husband. I sat in a trance, excusing myself to the bathroom periodically, during which time I'd pass blood clots and whatever small amount amniotic fluid had collected while I was lying prostrate. Nurses tracked my vital signs to keep watch for infection. My father-in-law offered us his space in the mausoleum next to my husband's mother, who had passed away five years earlier. At least she wouldn't be alone, we told ourselves.

My eyes remained swollen and raw from crying. I began to see in myself the same "bare life" described by Agamben's *zoē*. I had no words, no language. My body was an object to be measured and monitored. My hospital room door was marked with a white paper flower to notify workers tactfully that this was not a place to offer congratulations. They delivered food and towels silently, and I felt their pity. I was an asterisk, too. "Not this one," the little white flower would say.

While my family chatted and consoled, my thoughts turned into imagery, like a waking dream. My mind traced over my pregnancy story. I envisioned myself walking along a path in the woods. The forest floor was lined with gravel and dark roots tripping me up along the way. But I had somewhere to get to—a destination—so I kept walking forward. Then the path became level and I reached a clearing. I was going to make it, like so many women before me. I was going to be united with the person that I wanted to know, to care for. I was going to find her and we would bake cupcakes and I would make poorly constructed Halloween costumes for her so she could be whatever she wanted. I would despise her toys scattered on the floor, but I would love it, too. One foot in front of the other. Then, suddenly, there was a rupture, a great divide. The ground in front of me disappeared and there was no more forward. I was standing at the edge of a cliff with no path, no other side in sight. One more step and it would be over. I stood there, exposed, in the sun and wind. And though no one was around, I felt like I was being watched. It was Him. He was watching me, waiting for me to fall. I tried not to hate Him for it.

/

Somehow, in the forty-eight hours that followed, I did not go into active labor. Because I was unwilling to induce and technically stable, the new obstetrician on service discharged me on Monday morning. She made her opinion clear that we were choosing incorrectly, certain that labor would not hold off until the twenty-three-week mark when survival outside of the uterus would become remotely viable. She told us that we should be prepared to deliver the baby at home. I would have a check-up at my doctor's office on Wednesday if I made it that long. My mother came home with us to offer support and help my husband with the delivery if we couldn't make it back to the hospital in time.

Back at our apartment, I emailed our friends with the news, telling them that it would take a "miracle of miracles" for Zoey to survive. We tracked my temperature hourly and I kept my feet up. I drank cranberry juice as though that prevents infections, as though it would make a difference, though I knew it wouldn't. I stuck to my normal pregnancy diet, though my doctor had told me that it didn't matter anymore. I sang to Zoey in the shower like I had always done, wondering which bits of blood and tissue running down the drain were mine or hers. I tried to keep my belly in the sun when I could, sometimes lying on the carpet of our living room to catch the afternoon light. She had always seemed to like the warmth of it. I wasn't acting out of hope; I just wasn't ready to act like it was over. I wanted my time with her to be as good as possible. I wanted to be the mom I would have been if she could stay.

Still, my mind wandered. I found myself staring at the clock. "This minute, I'm more likely to go into labor than the last," I thought. And then I thought it all over again each time another minute ticked into the next. I thought about how quickly we could get to the hospital and noted that I should put extra lap pads in our travel bag so I wouldn't bleed all over my husband's car on the way. I thought about delivering at home and wondered if we would boil water (or whether people delivering term babies at home even do that anymore). I considered what we would do with Zoey's body, who would take her out of the toilet or wrap her up in towels on the bed. I didn't want my husband to see any of it or be a part of it. I didn't want him to hurt any more than necessary. I didn't want to share my shame.

I tried to numb myself with television. On several occasions, I found myself watching some movie depicting a triumph against the odds. As if on cue, Zoey would begin stirring inside of me. I couldn't help smiling. "Okay, you're still here," I thought, "I get it." Our situation was a fait accompli but every time I was about to accept it truly, she started kicking. I felt like she was giving me a nudge to hold on. In those moments, I thought, *Miracles happen and why not us.* Then I thought, *Miracles happen and why us.* I tried to breathe and focus on my love for her. I tried to channel it through my body so she could feel it, trusting that it was something of which we could both be certain.

/

Wednesday arrived and I returned to my obstetrician's office to see if anything had changed. The ultrasound technician took measurements; my cervix was normal but, as before, there was hardly any amniotic fluid left. The gestational sac hadn't healed over. Without more fluid around her, Zoey's lungs would not be able to develop. We hadn't achieved the critical step necessary for her to have a chance at survival. All the small traces of hope that had fought their way to the surface dissipated in the darkness of that room. I cried silently.

In a treatment room, my doctor confirmed that the prognosis was the same. She asked if I had thought any more about what I wanted to do. I realized that other people changed their minds about whether to induce labor, and I began to empathize with them. "I don't know," I said. Tears rolled out, speckling my shoes. "I just . . . I just don't want to give up on her," I explained. She assured me that no one could ever say I had given up and I noticed that her eyes were becoming wet. It was the first time I saw her become emotional.

In the end, she scheduled a consultation with a neonatologist to give us an idea of what to expect in case I made it to twenty-three weeks. But the referral came with a caution. We needed to keep in mind how unlikely it was that we'd make it that long, and how, in our case, Zoey's chances of survival were even smaller given the absence of fluid. We set up the appointment for the next day, still knowing there was every likelihood that I would go into labor before we set foot in the door.

We made it through the night, and the next morning, we met with the neonatologist. She was kind and supportive, but also direct. The survival rates in their neonatal intensive care unit were higher than I expected, with twenty-four-weekers having better than a 50 percent chance of survival. But she also explained that if Zoey did survive, every type of behavioral, cognitive, and physical impairment would be a possibility. She could be deaf, blind, or have cerebral palsy; she could require a ventilator or feeding tube for the rest of her life. The earlier she was born, the more likely she was to have more of these complications and the more severe each one would be. The likelihood of a problematic outcome was also exacerbated by the lack of fluid to help her lungs develop. The doctor was compassionate with us, saying that she understood if we chose to induce in that moment—many couples do.

As the meeting came to a close, I saw how much the lens through which I view the world was shaping my decision not to induce. My only sibling, a younger brother, has Down syndrome. I know enough not to underestimate the work and emotional challenge that can go into raising a child with special needs. But the prospect also didn't scare me or make me concerned about quality of life the same way it might for others. I thought about my Catholic upbringing and wondered how a woman raised in a progressive household might experience the same situation. I didn't expect the pain would necessarily be any different, but a part of me was almost jealous that someone else could have made a choice or felt some sense of control over the situation. I wasn't doing this to obey a religious rule, but my belief in a grand design must have informed my willingness to let our story of impending loss run its course. Maybe I was just too weak to let go. Choosing to induce would have seemed like the more merciful choice if she was going to suffer, be prodded and poked, and then pass away all the same.

I didn't know what to hope for anymore. I only knew I still wasn't ready to decide it was over.

Against the odds, I reached the twenty-three-week benchmark. I was admitted to the antepartum ward of the hospital with a Level 3 NICU. It was the same hospital that would have had the ability to induce labor just nine days earlier. I started to learn how important numbers would become in our medical team's decision-making. Since rupturing my membrane, my pregnancy had been counted in days, not weeks. Although a twenty-three-weeker was considered potentially viable, depending on her appearance, the doctors might not opt to resuscitate Zoey unless we gave them specific instructions to do so. They were also more likely to perform medical interventions for a baby weighing 500 grams or more because they have better survival rates.

I watched as the hospital's ultrasound technician struggled with the darkness of my uterus, trying to measure Zoey to estimate her weight. We were told that her weight was looking like 530 grams even before twenty-four weeks, so that was to our advantage. I marveled at the process. It was like a guessing game straining to achieve the appearance of precision. The kicker was that much of it relied on whether I had reported the first day of my last period correctly when I had found out I was pregnant four months earlier.

"I could have been wrong," I insisted. What if she was really two days further along in development than we thought? But she had been measuring close enough to expectation until that point, the doctors observed. I wanted to push back. Don't babies often measure somewhat small or large for gestation? I realized there was no point in arguing, so I tried to play the game to the best of my ability.

In our consultation with the neonatologist, we had been told that steroids could be given at twenty-three and a half weeks' gestation to encourage lung development. At first, it sounded like the godsend we had been looking for; up until that point, nobody had mentioned the potential to correct the absence of amniotic fluid. But, in our case, we were racing against the clock and there was still reason to expect I would go into labor before then. We were given the choice to administer the steroids early, but the doctors warned us that there was no data indicating they would work at this stage in the pregnancy. And we wouldn't be able to do a second round of steroids for three weeks. If Zoey were born in the interim, she could miss out on the benefit of the medication altogether. It was a gamble. Knowing that it would still take a period of time for the steroids to have an effect on her lungs, we decided to have them administered immediately.

As the nurse stuck the needle into my backside, I heard her murmur, "The things we do for love." I almost laughed aloud. I knew I'd take an injection every hour of every day for the rest of my life if it would improve Zoey's chances of surviving. I would cut off my finger if I could keep her. I wondered if there was some exchange rate of physical sacrifice that I didn't know about, some form of payment or punishment that would make this all go away. I stopped myself from going further down that road. In the Catholic telling, sacrifice is the ultimate expression of love. Sitting in a hospital bed, I saw how motherhood could give someone the capacity to love to the point of madness.

After spending nearly three weeks in that bed, I gave birth to Zoey at twenty-five weeks and three days' gestation. She weighed one pound and thirteen ounces. When her medical team finally stabilized her, a nurse was able to bring her over to me, just for a moment. The room was dim and she was bundled deep inside a nest of receiving blankets; I could barely make out her face. I touched her forehead gently with my thumb and told her I loved her. Then they rushed my baby away to the NICU. I wasn't sure I would ever see her again.

/

After eighty-six days in the hospital, Zoey came home with us. When I share this story with friends who have only known her as a child, they are shocked. They see that she is petite, but otherwise cannot imagine that she had this rough start in life. Oftentimes, they credit me for having hope, for not giving up on her. Almost always, they call her a miracle.

I leave these conversations feeling uncomfortable, like so many important things have gone unsaid. I didn't hang on to her because I had hope or faith. The truth is that I avoided feeling hopeful whenever possible. I just loved her. I just wanted to have every minute I could with her. If I lost her, I knew that I would torture myself for the rest of my life wondering if there was something more I could have done. So, I put in the time and work, yes. I spent every possible moment sitting by her bedside or holding her skin to skin. I pumped breastmilk as an obsessive labor of love, I attended rounds, and I left my job to give her the care she needed. And every day, I prayed. But having hope implies that I got the outcome I expected, that my faith was somehow rewarded. After my water broke just over halfway through a full-term pregnancy, the fact that she is a whole, functioning, happy child still regularly surprises me. I think there is a part of my life now that will always feel like a dream.

Some of my discomfort also stems from meeting families who have similar preemie stories and very different outcomes. In becoming involved in our NICU's advisory council, I met a couple whom I admire beyond words. Their daughter was a twenty-four-weeker who was beautiful, loved, and prayed for no less than my own. She graced this world for six months. In her memory, her parents have gone on to raise funds for equipment and to bring comfort to families in the NICU. They collaborate at a national level with medical professionals to improve patient care. In my heart, I know that I could not have shown this kind of strength and generosity in the midst of an enduring grief. It was not the outcome prayed for, hoped for ... but a light like theirs in the darkest of darkness? Well, *that* sure looks like a miracle to me. That is the grace of spirit where I see the greatest beauty of our humanity; that is where I see God.

Maybe my daughter is a miracle in the truest sense of the word. But if we honor her story primarily because of its amazing outcome, we not only diminish the value of the NICU babies who never make it home or who go home with extensive complications. We also fail to appreciate the core of Zoey's transition from the impossible to the possible. It wasn't just a magic trick. It was having an obstetrician who would educate and support me to make the best decision for myself. It was the neonatologists, nurses, and respiratory therapists who put in countless hours of study and practice, sacrificing time with their own families to save my own. It was the umbilical catheters, ventilators, and drug delivery systems developed by biomedical engineers in labs. It was blood donors whose politics and religion may be nothing like mine. It was the charitable women who sew blankets and knit tiny hats, giving families the dignity of being able to celebrate and comfort a new baby. It was my coworkers, some of whom I had never met, donating their paid sick time to me. It was the good fortune of our social class and my ability to stay by Zoey's side every day. It was our family and friends giving us a network of constant support. It was having a marriage that was caring and resilient—one that had already been tested by grief. Her life was fought for with hard work, scientific genius, generosity, compassion, and love.

And, for me, there was God. On my knees, I am grateful to God that I have Zoey in my life. I am grateful for every prayer uttered in her name—I needed every single one. Just as I needed every mind and hand that played a role in caring for her in our tangible world, I needed the divine. At the same time, I still wonder whether prayers are truly answered, or if they are only heard. I can't have it both ways, the logic goes. Either God saved her or He doesn't actually intervene. Either I believe He is real and thus real for everyone, or I don't. Either I look at Zoey as this miracle of miracles, or I look at every life, every outcome, as equally wondrous and valuable.

But it's not so simple. The most significant parts of our lives rarely are.

As much as I long to make sense of my faith and my experience of the preemie journey, there is something at the heart of it that logic and language misses. There is no such thing as infinity-plus-one, but that is how I love her every day—always increasing but never diminishing what came before. If having a micropreemie made me certain of anything, it is that there is a space for the impossible. Sometimes, that space is more meaningful, more accurate, than anything we can truly understand. My world centers around a life that was born from that space: our Zoey. I'm glad she's here.

Situationally Broke

BY ASHLEY FRANKLIN

It's easy to forget your financial situation when you've adapted to it. You're not hungry because you've learned how to stretch a meal. Rice isn't a side dish; it is a life-sustaining force that is an unmatched luxury once you learn how to vary its taste. You learn the value of a clearance rack and the best days to go thrifting. I was good at doing all of the things that helped me feel like a normal member of society—you know, not someone who is one missed paycheck away from homelessness. It was a false sense of security, but it was mine. No one could take that away from me. No one did, but something did: pregnancy.

I found out I was pregnant about a month after I stopped taking the pill. It was sooner than my husband and I had expected, but we were still excited. Something else I hadn't expected was that the pregnancy made me eligible for Medicaid. Suddenly, I had a couple of choices for where I could receive my prenatal checkups, and the clinic I chose seemed like the better option. I'm still not sure if I was right, but I followed my gut—the gut of a broke, young African American woman who was having her first child hundreds of miles away from her family and who was panicked at the idea of anything less than a perfect birth experience.

Why was I so panicked? Because photos of me connected to bundles of wires have been emblazoned in my mind for as long as I can remember. You see, I was a preemie. And if going to the clinic to ensure I had proper prenatal care was the answer to all my fears, then there was no question that's what I would do. I could no longer afford to hold onto the delusion that I wasn't poor enough to need Medicaid. My high horse had turned into a low pony, and I was fine with that. I was going to do whatever it took to have a normal, stress-free pregnancy.

The clinic was located on the third floor of a hospital in Monroe, Louisiana. There was a large waiting area with several rows of fake individual chairs—you know, the chairs that looked separate but were actually connected. They gave you a false sense of autonomy. Connecting all the chairs was genius because it prevented patients from picking up individual chairs and hurling them at the large glass windows—something I thought about doing at least twice an appointment. That sounds irrational now, but it seemed like a perfectly rational way to relieve my stress and frustration after waiting there for hours each nerve-wracking visit before even getting my vitals checked.

But during those initial months of pregnancy, I learned to apply the golden rule of getting ahead: It's not what you know. It's who you know. I got to know every nurse, assistant, and greeter that I could. I didn't know it at the time, but every connection I made in that clinic would soon overlap with the connections I'd made just a few months earlier at the local masjid when I converted to Islam.

And connections like these are what kept me and my preemie alive when I was unexpectedly diagnosed with preeclampsia. My blood pressure was high, my hands and feet were abnormally swollen, and there was protein in my urine. None of these things had been apparent just one month earlier. It was the biggest unwanted surprise of my life, considering preeclampsia could end up killing me and the baby if left unchecked.

At twenty-five, I didn't know much about my family's medical history. My mother knew little more than I did. We gathered that high blood pressure and diabetes runs in our family—though I hadn't had issues with either. We also agreed that I hadn't been a sickly child, aside from my early start. But I didn't need to rely on my mother's knowledge to know the flashing lights and sounds coming from the machine taking my blood pressure couldn't be good. It was February 15. I was days shy of being thirty weeks pregnant, and with a blood pressure reading of 150/100, I was admitted to the hospital after what should have been a regular prenatal visit.

Fortunately, I had a first line of defense against the feelings of inadequacies and fault I began to feel: those nurses, assistants, and greeters I'd befriended during my months at the clinic. That brigade of Black women who referred to me as "Baby" at every prenatal appointment now took care of me and helped stave off the inevitable guilt and stress over the turn my pregnancy had taken. And then help arrived in the middle of the night during my twenty-four-hour observation time. She had only one question: "What are you doing here and why didn't you tell me?"

Let's call her Dr. I. I'd met her at the masjid—and more importantly, she was the head of anesthesiology. She had clout. She immediately notified the other doctors from the masjid who worked at the hospital that I was there. Dr. I offered me peace of mind, but after asking how the other doctors were treating me, she also offered this piece of advice: "Make sure to tell them that you know me."

And that's just what I did. Everything changed with the doctors and nurses who were in and out of my room. They became extra accommodating. When shifts changed or when an additional medical person entered the room, they did the name dropping for me.

"This is Mrs. Franklin. She's a friend of Dr. I's. Make sure she's well taken care of."

What kind of care was I getting before? This is a question that lingered in the back of my mind. I'm not saying I was treated poorly before, but I can say I was now treated differently. Maybe this new connection added an extra sense of accountability on their part. Maybe they were afraid I would say something negative and it would get back to a superior. I don't know. All I know is I felt like I'd been chosen—not in the holy-light-with-an-angelic-soundtrack type of way, but more like a claw-machine-rescue type of way. Dr. I reminded me that I deserved to be treated just like any other patient.

At the end of my twenty-four-hour watch, I was told the hospital staff wouldn't be able to adequately care for my baby at the facility. The preeclampsia diagnosis was confirmed. My blood pressure remained high, and there was an abundance of protein in my urine. I had two choices:

Option 1: Stay at this hospital to give birth and then let them take my preemie to a hospital with a more advanced neonatal intensive care unit located a couple of hours away.

Option 2: Go to that hospital now.

I chose Option 2.

/

Two hours and one bumpy ambulance ride later, I was at a new hospital in Shreveport.

Being at Shreveport was different. It was also a teaching hospital, but it was bigger, had more resources, and seemed better equipped to handle low-income and under- or uninsured people with complex health issues. But, perhaps because of that, many of the doctors I encountered presented a worse bedside manner than back in Monroe. I felt like I was seen as yet another textbook example of a poor person whose negligence with their health landed them in a bad situation. It made those who had listened to me and who had treated me with genuine kindness and concern during my first hospital stay all the more precious.

But these weren't my doctors. And this wasn't my town. My pregnancy had robbed me of everything—including but not limited to my health. In less than forty-eight hours, I'd lost every ounce of security I should have had. Each trip in and out of the triage department made me feel like I was losing the connection with the tiny human inside of me. Nothing about this pregnancy was normal. Shuffling between triage and my hospital bed as my legs and feet morphed into puffy, unrecognizable masses was my new normal. Frankly, I was over it.

Every conversation with the doctors went the same way.

"You must have a history of high blood pressure," they would say.

"No, I don't," I'd respond, getting wearier each time.

"Well, how do you know if you haven't had proper care?"

"Because I'm poor, not an idiot."

Here I was with a master's degree, having people think I wasn't smart enough to take care of my health. That wasn't the case at all. I'd always taken care of myself, even when I wasn't able to afford health care on my own. But you can swing a cat and hit five millennials with advanced degrees and zero financial stability these days; I was certainly not the only one to fall into the health care gap.

I went to a wonderful liberal arts college for my bachelor's degree, majoring in the humanities. I'd actually started off as pre-med. It may seem odd that I'd jump from pre-med to English, but trust me: I did the world a favor. I was terrible at organic chemistry. I tried out several majors in between, hoping to land on one I enjoyed that wouldn't leave me broke. As hard as I fought it, I ended up following the age-old advice to do what I loved and the rest would come together. I was smart, even when I wasn't wise. I followed my love of literature into a master's program. I was going to be a college professor! At least, that was the plan until I was three-quarters of the way through my program and realized I didn't like the atmosphere of academia. This left me uniquely overqualified to do nothing; I'd only ever had academic jobs for my entire life. Out of countless applications submitted, there were only two places willing to hire me: Toys "R" Us (may they rest in peace) and a daycare. I went with the daycare because they were willing to pay me $1 more—a whopping $9 an hour. Still, I had bills to pay, so I pieced together freelance gigs and wrote for content mills. I was living proof that not everyone with a master's degree raked in the dough.

So, no. I have never had consistent health care, not even in childhood. But I did seek care when it was needed, and I was able to get yearly physicals—and I had perfectly normal blood pressure at each one, thank you very much. It just wasn't as easy as scheduling a doctor's appointment whenever I wanted. Now, I was thankful for the government program that funded prenatal health care during pregnancy. I was a patient who was on Medicaid, not just a Medicaid patient.

But that didn't seem to matter to anyone else. According to the doctors, I was someone who had neglected her health, and this was the result. Everything that was happening to me, and to the baby I was about to deliver, was my fault.

I'm not just assuming this is what the doctors thought, battling with them in my head years later over perceived slights and bruised egos. I know it's what they thought because they said it out loud on rounds. I was at a teaching hospital, and I heard the doctors explain to the residents: "You see this woman? She is very sick and has been sick for a long time due to high blood pressure."

I wanted to fight back, to tell the doctors that they didn't even know me. But I knew my situation was too precarious. I couldn't get unnecessarily snarky with folks who could potentially save my life. And I was on my way to having a preemie.

At *my* hospital, I had already received a shot to help develop my baby's lungs faster than normal in the event of his early arrival. My village had made sure of that. I was in Shreveport now—not my town, not my people, but I was NOT going to get through this without them. Clearly, I was going to need all the help I could get. That wasn't going to happen without any allies. I dug deep—I'm talking bottom of my marshmallow-puffed feet deep—for the most pleasant personality I could find. I could no longer wish for the warmth I'd felt from the Black community of honorary aunties or rely on the connections of who I knew from the masjid. It was up to me to create a safe, validating space with whatever kind souls I could at the new hospital.

I did what needed to be done. I found a new group of people—nurses and doctors and other caregivers at the hospital—but my husband remained at its core. He was an enormous source of strength and was a trooper through it all. His day job was flexible, but he was also attending school at night. Both were a significant distance from the hospital. He stayed with me as much as he could, doing his best to keep my spirits high—aside from repeatedly kicking my butt at Uno. My in-laws, particularly my mother-in-law, showed up like the blessed waymakers they were—even bringing a diaper bag loaded with goodies. It's funny. I'd had so much planned out, including the specific diaper bag I wanted. Now, none of that mattered. That Walmart diaper bag was packed with more than stuff; it was packed with love. The green-and-brown bag with the odd-looking giraffe on it made a big statement: someone else believed that everything was going to be okay.

I wasn't due until April, and the doctors told me that I would remain in the hospital until I delivered. They wanted me to reach at least thirty-two weeks, but longer would be ideal. I was already tired of hospitals. The thought of remaining there for possibly months was too much to bear. I pulled out my ace in the hole. I called my cousin, an obstetrician in a different state. She helped me to understand what the doctors were doing and saying in layman's terms. She gave it to me straight and told me the doctors were trying to prolong my delivery as long as they could to give the baby a chance to develop more. (Have you ever really wanted a family member to be wrong?) After our conversation, I was convinced. I was going to ride out the rest of my pregnancy like a champ.

As fate would have it, I wouldn't be dealing with those frustrations for long. Why? Two weeks was all my body (and the baby) could handle. I was getting worse. The baby's oxygen levels were too erratic. Ladies and gentlemen, this show was over at thirty-two weeks. And like any decent show, the finale came with a surprise twist—my mother flew in from Delaware. We may have come up short with our family's medical history, but Mom showed up big when it mattered most. Like any mother/daughter duo with very similar personalities, we tend to clash . . . a lot. But we didn't have time for that. We had bigger—or, rather, smaller—matters of great importance to tackle. My mother's tough-love approach snapped me out of "woe is me" and planted me firmly into "handle your business" territory. She had been through this before. I was her preemie, and here I was with a preemie of my own. Life, huh?

I was at my most vulnerable just before meeting the tiniest, most vulnerable baby I'd ever had the privilege of holding. Bilal weighed two pounds, ten ounces when he was born. I felt unworthy to hold him. It was terrifying. He was layered in blankets, yet I could barely feel his weight in my arms. No matter. The responsibility of caring for someone so fragile and not knowing how long he'd have to be in the NICU alone were weighing heavily on me. I was filled to the brink with a fearful hope. Life gave me a preemie while simultaneously stripping me of nearly everything that made me feel safe and secure. But I learned that there are other kinds of security. There are people who will always show up to fight for you and with you. For me, it was the hospital staff, Dr. I, my family, and my brand-new son.

I may have misspoken earlier. I was never poor. I couldn't have been with the amount of love and support I received from so many people. I was rich beyond measure. I was just situationally broke.

You're So Lucky

BY SUZANNE KAMATA

Dr. Nakagawa (Dr. "In the River," you translate in your head) is the man who's supposed to keep your children alive. When you first see him, the word that pops into your head is "young." He has brush-cut hair and dimples. His ample belly strains against the pink smock. From the back, you can see that he's wearing a T-shirt underneath—casual clothes when professionalism would seem to dictate button-downs and neckties. Get my babies out of here, you think. You'll take them to the Citizen's Hospital on the other side of the city, to gray-templed physicians and decades of experience. But then you see that your newborn twins are trussed up with wires and tubes. The long thin tube going into each tiny mouth conveys oxygen to their lungs. Minuscule IV needles are threaded into their veins. There are wires linking heartbeats to monitors. Those babies aren't going anywhere. You'll have to trust this man.

/

Japan, the country you have lived in for ten years, never felt so foreign as it did on the day when you were forced to check into one of its hospitals.

"Threatened premature labor," the doctor told you, and you gasped because you were only six months pregnant.

You had been planning on starting a program of Mozart and poetry in the seventh month, had already picked out a layette in the Lands' End mail-order catalog. You had just started wearing maternity clothes and ordered a gray cotton dress that hadn't even arrived yet. You had an appointment the next week with a doula recommended by your hippie friend who lives in the mountains.

According to your pregnancy diary, the lungs had not yet fully developed. Your babies' eyes were still closed. The ultrasound indicated that one of your unborn babies was less than a pound, the other barely over two.

/

Most Japanese women go back to their childhood homes to give birth. They spend the early weeks of motherhood in the rooms where they first dreamed of bouquet-bearing suitors and careers in film. Their husbands go to work and make phone calls at night.

You wanted to stay near your husband, and besides, your insurance wouldn't cover childbirth in another country. You'd picked out a small ladies' clinic locally famous for its good food (ice cream bars every afternoon, celebratory red snapper right after the baby is born). The rooms have floral curtains and you can almost pretend you're staying at a cozy bed-and-breakfast instead of a hospital.

You settle in with a stack of novels and a collection of silk bed jackets. Your Japanese mother-in-law shows up every day with cream puffs and freshly laundered pajamas. She sits by your bed for hours, long after you have run out of things to say to one another.

You read, you eat, you have exams. And then the doctor tells you that you must leave. The bleeding has not abated. You'd be better off in the ward of a bigger hospital—one with incubators and a neonatal intensive care unit.

"I like it here," you protest. "And I like you."

The doctor shakes his head. "No. You should go."

Two hospitals nearby are equipped to care for premature babies. One is a teaching hospital boasting the latest techniques and machinery; the other is the Citizen's Hospital. While you don't relish the idea of med students traipsing in and out of your room, in the end you have no choice. There are no beds available in the maternity ward of the other hospital.

So you are transferred by ambulance, sirens singing you along the highway. Because you are horizontal, you cannot see the other cars making way.

/

Your mother has never seemed as far away as she does on the day you are rushed into the operating theater. A few weeks of bed rest have suddenly turned into blood running down your legs and an emergency Cesarean, and you are desperate for the safe and familiar.

Fortunately, your husband is only a phone call away. He arrives shortly after the obstetrician, who was called in on a Saturday, still in his day-off clothes—a striped polo shirt and khakis. You see your husband long enough to tell him that you are sorry about the failure of your body to keep the babies inside. You tell him about the pain that feels as if it is cracking you apart. You press your wedding ring into his palm and then you are wheeled away.

The nurses in white run with the gurney down one corridor and the next, into a darker part of the hospital that is unfamiliar to you. There, you are handed off to another set of nurses and they take you the rest of the way.

On the operating table, you are surrounded by strangers wearing blue gauze masks and matching smocks. You look at the clock: 5:30 a.m.

The nurse tells you to curl into a ball and you do and the

needle slides into your spine. You wonder if you'll be able to speak Japanese under anesthesia.

You'd expected childbirth to be something else entirely—Enya on the stereo, champagne chilling in the hospital mini-fridge, your husband's fingers kneading the small of your back. Instead, he is in another room and the obstetrician is swabbing and slicing your abdomen. There is a screen between you and the action so you can't see a thing. You feel liquid ooze and gush, and the hands of the doctor reaching into your womb. There is movement, like a fish flopping against your belly, and then a tiny mewling cry.

"*Kawaii*," the doctor says. "Cute." But you can only imagine, because your son is immediately whisked off to an incubator before you can catch a glimpse of him.

"Now we're going in for the other one," the doctor says, and he reaches for the girl who has lived beneath your heart for the past few months. And then she is taken away, too, and the worst part is over. Or so you think.

/

Your mother-in-law arrives for her daily visit before your husband has a chance to call her with the news. You hear the rustle of plastic bags filled with oranges and yogurt and then you hear her gasp. When you open your eyes, you see that she is looking at you as if you are dying.

You have never been so thirsty in your life, but the nurses say "No drinking or eating." Your legs are still numb from the anesthesia. When your mother-in-law pours you a cup of juice and urges you to drink, you have to remind yourself that it's a gesture of kindness, not torture.

Over the next few days and weeks you will spend more time with your mother-in-law than anyone else.

/

You enter the NICU for the first time the following evening, nearly a day and a half after the twins' birth. The first time you see your babies, see the swell of their eyeballs under sealed eyelids, you think "baby bird." And then you look at their thin, bowed legs and think "bullfrog." Their heads, so narrow, so large in proportion to their bodies: aliens.

They have little beards, but no eyelashes. You can't make out the shapes of their mouths, which are taped to the breathing tubes.

Your husband was right. They do not look like the babies on the covers of your magazines, but you are wrenched with a violent kind of love. If you could will them back into your body, you would. You are sorry you dreaded the pain of childbirth. Let them tear you apart if they could be born again, healthy.

/

The NICU nurses' photos are tacked to the wall. In several of the snapshots, the nurses are holding the pale-skinned black-haired baby next to your son's incubator. He is a giant—six or seven pounds at least. Your son weighs less than two pounds.

The nurse in charge of your boy is Ms. Matsumoto. She goes about her work with the enthusiasm of a kindergarten teacher. She dances with the giant baby to the tune of Brahms's "Lullaby" and takes him for "walks." She reaches into your son's incubator and waves his hand around as if he were an action figure. "Genki da yo!" she says in a baby boy's voice. "Don't worry! I'm fine!"

Sometimes Nurse Matsumoto teases Dr. Nakagawa. This seems bizarre in a country where authority demands respect.

You wonder if they are flirting, even though there is no word for "flirt" in the Japanese language. Most of the NICU staff is young and you wonder if they have affairs with each other like the nurses and doctors in the TV show *ER*. You wonder if they are married. No rings are allowed in the NICU so it's difficult to tell. No watches, either. Everyone must wear a pink smock over their clothes (pink being a color found to be soothing to babies), a white cap over their hair. The parents wear masks. You have to wash your hands three times before you can touch your babies.

/

Every three hours, you and the other new parents go to the Nipple Room. It's not really called that; it has some Japanese name that you can never remember, but the Nipple Room seems more apt.

All five or six of you (the number varies) sit on cushioned benches with your pajamas unbuttoned and your pink or brown nipples bared. There is none of the modesty that you've experienced in women's locker rooms in Japan. You compare and admire each others' breasts.

"Mine are so hard," one woman moans. "Feel them."

At her urging, you press the pads of your fingers against her swollen breast and indeed, it is solid.

When the nurse hands over her giant baby boy, she tickles his parted lips with her nipple, but he won't suck.

"Don't sleep," she says. "Give me some relief."

You are jealous that she has a baby to suckle even if he is reluctant. You sit there beside her, eking colostrum from your own breasts. It slides into the sterilized bottle, thick and yellow, drop by precious drop. Your fingers ache. Your lily white breasts are stained with bruises.

You've heard that thoughts of babies activate the ducts, make the milk flow faster, so you think about your son and daughter.

Your boy has a slender tube through his nose which goes directly to his stomach. Every two hours, he is fed two milli liters of your milk. Two cubic centimeters—that's maybe a teardrop, or as much dew as falls on one leaf of clover.

This morning when you sat before your daughter's incubator listening to the hum of the respirator, Dr. Nakagawa told you that she could not digest the milk. Although she, too, was fed through a tube from nose to stomach, the colostrum remains in her stomach, unprocessed. The feeding will be stopped. If she can't eat, how will she stay alive?

/

"I've heard that physical contact can make all the difference with preemies," your college roommate emails from New York.

You've heard that too, but you're afraid to touch your babies. You open the Plexiglas doors to your daughter's incubator and stroke her foot with one finger. She jerks away.

"I'm your mother," you whisper sadly. "I'm giving you affection."

Her eyes are still sealed shut. She cannot look at you.

You caress her arms, ever so lightly, and then her head, and then brush your fingertips over her torso. The monitor alarm goes off. You look up quickly and then snatch your hand away when you see that her heart rate has suddenly dropped from 112 beats per minute to 60.

A nurse comes running toward you, rubber soles squeaking on the floor, and then Dr. Nakagawa.

"You'd better let her rest for a while," he says. Then he smiles sadly, as if to assure you that it wasn't entirely your fault.

/

Your mother-in-law arrives with bags of souvenirs. She has spent the previous evening preparing packages of little bean-filled cakes, oranges, and iron-supplemented soft drinks for the visitors sure to stream into your room.

"It's the seventh day," she says knowingly. "And an auspicious day on the calendar."

There is still so much that you don't know about local tradition, but you are quite sure that no well-wishers will arrive. Later, you will learn that the people in the office where you worked are wondering if your babies are even alive.

It is hard to decide if this is a celebratory occasion or not.

Your parents send a bouquet of flowers and a card saying "Thank you for our new grandchildren."

You aunt calls from Michigan and her first words are "I'm so sorry."

Your mother-in-law, who has not yet seen the babies, knows only that you have provided an heir. She sits by your bed all day and puts on her social smile every time the door opens, but it is only the cleaning lady come to scrub the toilet, the handsome young intern to change your IV fluid, the nurse to take your temperature, a mischievous child who barged into the wrong room.

When your husband arrives that evening to spell her, your mother-in-law's face is heavy and sad. All of the bags that she has brought remain in a corner of the room.

/

A couple of days later—an unlucky day according to your mother-in-law's calendar—your hippie friend comes to visit.

The nurse, with her finger to your pulse, studies him out of the corner of her eye. What must she think of this pony-tailed man in a poet's blouse? Does she think that this is an assignation, a tryst? He has arrived with a tattered paperback of Anne Waldman under one arm and a bowl of salad in the other.

The nurse finishes her business and leaves, and you lay against the white sheets while he feeds you freshly picked parsley, spinach, and sprouts on a fork.

You tell him about the treatment that your children are getting.

Your hippie friend who self-medicates with herbal teas says, "All those chemicals can't be good for them."

But you know that without them, your babies would die.

/

There is one other woman who expresses milk by hand. Her newborn son (1,318 grams and growing) is in the NICU, too. His incubator is next to your baby girl's.

One day you start talking about mothers-in-law.

"My mother-in-law," you say, "sits by my bed all day. I just want to read my book, but I feel as if I should entertain her."

"My mother-in-law," you say, "is always hovering and fussing. If I so much as cough, she jumps up to throw a blanket over me even though I'm sweating. It drives me nuts."

"Mine never visits," the other woman says.

"Why not?"

"Because she blames me for this." And you know that she is referring to her own bum womb and the tiny boy behind Plexiglas.

On another day, you hear a nurse tell a story of a woman who was divorced for giving birth to a stillborn child. The husband and mother-in-law discussed it while the wife was still convalescing, still grappling with her grief, no doubt. They gave her the news the day after she was released from the hospital.

You realize that the woman who annoys you so much is not so bad after all.

/

You walk into the NICU in your mask and smock and paper hat and the young doctor motions you to his desk.

"Your son is fine," he says. "No problem."

And then he takes out a photo done by ultrasound, shows you the blue spots that indicate blood in your daughter's lungs. He draws a picture of the heart's chambers and scratches words above it: "ductus arteriosis." It seems that a duct in your daughter's heart has failed to close as it should have after birth. Her body has not adapted to life outside the womb; her lungs don't understand that they must now fill with oxygen.

The doctor tells you that there is medication and, if that doesn't work, they can try surgery. He gives you a form to sign your consent.

You sit by her incubator longer than usual.

"My little sweet pea," you say. "My darling girl."

She weighs no more than a small animal—a squirrel, perhaps, or a chipmunk. You cannot imagine such a delicate being surviving cuts and sutures.

When you go back to your room, your mother-in-law is there, plumping pillows and changing the water in the vases of flowers—flowers for "congratulations" and "get well soon."

You try to smile, but your spirits are flagging. You show her the form explaining the problem and the procedure for dealing with your baby girl's heart. It is all in Japanese. You explain as well as you can that there is a duct that needs to be closed. You try to be brave and confident because you know how much your mother-in-law will worry if you aren't.

The next day when you visit your children, Dr. Nakagawa is

listening to opera in his office. You can hear Italians warbling through the partition and you try to identify the music. A tragedy? A comedy? Is this one of those stories where the heroine dies consumptive at the end?

The other four babies in the NICU have been released from their Plexiglas prisons. They are given suck at intervals by cheerful moms, taken on promenades by the nurses, bathed in the stainless-steel sink. If Dr. Nakagawa is worried, it's because of your children. It's because of the baby girl balanced between heaven and life on earth.

But then the young doctor emerges from his haven and smiles.

"Your son," he says, "no problem."

"And my daughter?"

"Getting better."

Yesterday's tears were tears of fear and sorrow and worry, but today's are something else altogether.

On the fourth day, the ultrasound reveals that the duct has closed completely. The treatment was a success.

You are exhausted from midnight and three and six a.m. milkings, from the heart-pumping drama you've been forced to endure, from the bedside hovering of your mother-in-law. When you find her, once again plumping pillows, changing water, rearranging toiletries and so on, you explain in your best Japanese that the duct in your daughter's heart has closed. And then you tell her that you want to take a nap. She nods gravely and leaves you alone in the shuttered room.

You sleep. When your mother-in-law returns an hour later, you see that she has been crying. She tells you that she has been wandering the hospital halls worrying about your baby girl.

"The duct closed," you say. "It's a *good* thing."

/

So now your daughter is getting better. She is being fed breast milk. She is growing stronger.

But then the doctor tells you that although the duct in your son's heart closed on its own, it has now reopened.

"That can happen?" you ask.

"Yes, sometimes. But rarely."

You feel helpless, much like you do when an earthquake rocks your house. Everything is unpredictable, subject to chance.

You are given another form to sign. On this day you sit next to your son's incubator longer than usual.

/

On the day that you come home from the hospital, ten days after the birth of your children, your next-door neighbor is weeding her flower bed. She sees you get out of the car with your little brown suitcase. She looks from your face to your diminished stomach, wipes her hands on her pants, and ambles over.

"Congratulations," she says. "A boy and a girl at once. You're so lucky."

Your neighbor had a baby when she was just this side of forty, after years of trying. She has a five-year-old girl and from what she's implied, there'll be no more children. There is an aura of envy around her.

"They're still in the hospital," you say. "They're on life support."

She waves away your concern. "They'll be fine. These days incubators are just like the mother's womb."

You reflect upon this. Inside, the body is warm and dark. The incubator is a brightly lit space. Sometimes the nurses wrap gauze around your babies' feet and hands because their extremities chill easily. Inside the body, babies are lulled by the mother's heartbeat and the sound of her voice. The NICU is a cacophony of alarms and beeps and buzzes and infants screaming in pain.

/

After you leave the hospital, everyone you run into asks "Why?" Why did you go into premature labor? Why were your babies born fourteen weeks early?

Your older woman friend thinks it's because you let your legs get cold. She saw you at a musical in February in a knee-length dress and nothing but nylons when you should have been wearing insulated pants.

Your boss believes it's because you walked to work each day—a five-minute saunter, if that—carrying a soft-sided briefcase containing notebooks and a magazine or two. He doesn't consider that the cigarette smoke perpetually fogging the office might have had something to do with it. You have a flashback to a cup of coffee downed at your desk in the third month and you wonder if that might be it.

Your husband thinks it's because you went to an African dance party the week before you started to bleed. You knew when you walked to the bus stop and, later, when you boarded the train that your husband wouldn't approve. But he was in Hokkaido on business, and you would have been alone. Better to be among caring friends, you'd thought.

Maybe you shouldn't have moved the furniture when your husband called and said, "The new recliner will be delivered in ten minutes. Clear out a space."

But then you think about your sister-in-law who traveled to Bolivia on business in her seventh month of pregnancy, who rested her wine glass on the shelf of her stomach in between sips of Chardonnay, who actually went jogging until a few days before giving birth. Her son, your nephew, was born after two hours of labor.

Who is the freak of nature? You or your sister-in-law? And how can something so ordinary, so natural, go so wrong?

/

The giant baby is transferred from the NICU to the floor above, to pediatrics. On the day of his departure, you watch his mother dress him in striped blue pajamas. She packs up his stuffed bear and the mobile that played Brahms's "Lullaby" loud enough for the other babies to hear, and then they are gone.

In a few days the doctor will try to take the tube out of your daughter's lungs.

/

Without the tube, you can see that your daughter's mouth is shaped like Clara Bow's. It's a beautiful mouth. Until now, she has sucked on the tube for solace, but now she gapes like a fish out of water.

"Her mouth is lonely," the nurse says.

You wish you could slide your pinky between her lips.

For the first few hours, she takes regular breaths on her own. But in the days that follow, she sometimes forgets to inhale. When she stops breathing, the monitor beeps. You step aside quickly to allow the nurse to reach in and jiggle her. After a moment, her chest rises and falls, and you start breathing again, too. It takes a while to get used to it, but you do. Soon, you are the one to reach in and remind her to breathe.

/

You are singing to your daughter, making up the words as you go along: "My darling child, my little peanut, my ballerina girl."

Suddenly, the doors whoosh open. In comes the young doctor, a flock of nurses, and a pair of incubators. Another set of twins has been born, alas, too early. You stop singing and sit frozen like a bird in the bush.

The doctor calls out for things and the nurses hand them over. Each baby is weighed. Within five minutes, both red-skinned newborns are intubated and set up with IVs. You admire the staff's brisk competence. This must be what it was like on the day of your babies' birth.

The new twins, you notice, two boys, are slightly larger than your son was at birth. Your daughter remains the smallest patient in the NICU. You want to seek out the parents and tell them that you know how they feel.

"But look!" you'd say. "Our boy was smaller still and now he thrives!"

His mouth twitches in a smile. His hand curls around your finger.

The mother is wheeled in on a gurney, up close to the incubators. You watch her reach inside to touch each one and think, "How lucky! I had to wait till I was able to walk by myself to see my children."

But then the heart specialist is called in. He and the other doctors confer behind screens. They speak in hushed tones to the twins' parents.

When you visit two days later, one of the new twins is missing. In its place is an incubator covered with vinyl.

You know that it is none of your business, but you gesture and ask, "What happened to the other one?"

The nurse frowns at you with your bad manners. She makes a stalling sound—"mmmm"—and you lower your eyes.

"Oh," you say. "Pardon me."

In that same week, another baby dies and your daughter's kidneys stop functioning.

/

Your daughter's face is puffy with water; her diapers remain dry. Two days ago, she was delicate and slender. Now, the nurses joke that she looks like a sumo wrestler.

"We've never seen anything like this before," Dr. Nakagawa tells you. "In most cases, kidney failure occurs immediately after birth, not two months later."

"What's causing it?" you ask.

He answers with the most chilling words yet: "We don't know."

This is a country where doctors pretend to be gods, a condition which makes his frankness all the more alarming. For once in your life, you would have preferred a lie, some fake confidence.

When milk time comes around, your daughter gets nothing. She is being fed intravenously until her condition improves.

/

The doctor tells you that your son is almost ready to go home. You have nearly forgotten that these days will end, that you are the true guardian of the baby boy and girl in the incubators. The thought of taking care of them by yourself—the responsibility— terrifies you.

You are sitting, watching your daughter's miniature chest rise and fall, when you see something black out of the corner of your eye. It's a fly. You think, at first, that it's in the incubator with your baby, but then you notice that it's crawling up the blinds.

"Hey!" you call out, in a panic. "There's a fly in here!"

Flies carry germs. Flies cause African Sleeping Sickness and other diseases that could kill your children.

One of the nurses, the one who is always impeccably made-up, strolls over. "Where?" she asks. Her voice is calm.

You point to the winged vermin now exploring the top of your daughter's incubator.

The nurse takes a rolled-up notebook and swats. The fly is dead. You breathe a sigh of relief.

"How'd it get in here?" you ask. The windows are sealed.

"It must have followed one of you mothers in here," she says. "Maybe it likes the smell of your milk."

A couple days later, when you go to another part of the hospital for insurance purposes, you see a kitten in the corridor. A kitten: fleas, mites, toxoplasmosis.

"Nurse," you call out to a young woman in starched white. "There's a cat in here!"

The nurse looks in the direction you are waving in.

"So there is," she says with a smile. "How cute!" And then, believe it or not, she walks away, off to the ladies' room.

You wonder if you are being paranoid. You wonder if you will be able to protect your son—and later your daughter—from all the black flies and kittens and other dangers in the world.

/

Your son begins breathing room air, unassisted. He is taken out of the incubator and installed in a Plexiglas bed. He starts drinking breast milk from a bottle and then, little by little, from your breast. He cries loudly whenever he is hungry, and you worry that he might be disturbing the other babies who are weaker and sicker.

Dr. Nakagawa tells you that when your baby boy reaches 2,500 grams, he can go home. He now tips the scale at 2,300.

You haven't finished preparing the nursery yet, but this news brings a bloom to your cheeks. It's been almost three months since he departed your body and you long to have him close again.

Dr. Nakagawa asks you if you'd like to schedule his release for an auspicious day on the Japanese calendar. You are not superstitious like your mother-in-law, but you know that she would be horrified if your son left the NICU on an unlucky day. You are not superstitious, but you are willing to take all the help you can get.

/

The medicine that the doctors prescribed for your daughter has worked. Her kidneys are functioning properly once again and her second chin has melted. Her milk intake is increased. She is getting better, but you take nothing for granted. There have been too many surprises along the way. Every day your husband chants Buddhist sutras and you pray to another deity while on your knees.

A couple weeks later, your daughter begins to acquire the suggestion of meat around her thighs. At last, she grows eyelashes.

/

By the day that your son is ready to check out of the hospital, your tiny baby girl is out of the incubator as well, engulfed in a gauze kimono and swaddled in a white bath towel.

You dress your son in baby clothes for the first time. The little sailor outfit is intended for a preemie, but it is roomy on your boy.

You and your husband give the NICU staff a box of cream puffs and a case of soft drinks as an infinitesimal token of your appreciation. Insurance has pretty much picked up the tab for your children's care, but you want to pay back something.

Everyone gathers round as you prepare to take your boy out. You can't speak because your throat is jammed shut by emotion. Instead, you bow and let the doctors and nurses see the tears in your eyes.

You hold your daughter a little longer than usual on this day. She looks up at you with clear gray eyes. You wonder if she will notice that her brother, her wombmate, is no longer in the next bed, and if she will cry out in the night. Twins belong together, you think, but for now, they must separate. When she has closed her eyes and drifted into sleep, you force yourself to put her down until tomorrow morning. You don't know this yet, but your daughter will be released from the hospital in another month, when the nights begin to cool and the leaves begin to crisp.

You tuck your son into a wicker basket with a comforter printed in a teddy bear motif. Then you carry him out the whooshing door. When you step onto the elevator with your baby-boy-in-a-basket, it feels like you are doing something illegal.

You can now hold, feed, and bathe your son whenever you want to. The nurses no longer have any say. Dr. Nakagawa's work is done. Now it's up to you to keep him alive.

Outside, cars and trucks drive past. The grass is green. Swallows swoop overhead and the sound of giggles floats over from a nearby kindergarten. It's late summer and the sun is shining on your child for the first time.

What Genetics Research Doesn't Prepare You For: Premature Twins

BY DAN KOBOLDT

My daughter was born perfectly healthy at full term (thirty-seven weeks). Beyond the normal first-baby stresses, the experience was a sheer delight. So a year and a half later, when we learned my wife was pregnant, we felt confident. After all, we had *done* the baby thing. We had the equipment in hand: everything from bibs to wipe warmers. The infant car seat hadn't yet expired, and our small SUV should provide more than enough room for the four of us.

We also had firsthand parenting knowledge and skills, something no amount of books or classes can replace. We had changed hundreds, if not thousands, of diapers. We knew how to bathe, feed, burp, and swaddle an infant, a formula that resulted in our daughter sleeping for long stretches before the six-month mark. My wife and I were a good team, and, as we reassured one another after we learned she was pregnant, we'd still have one-on-one coverage. We could handle it.

Nature has a way of taking overconfident parents down a peg or two. Your baby's finally sleeping five hours at night? It's teething time. You think you've mastered diapers? Try this category-five blowout! These comeuppances are some of the Great Joys of Parenting. I've had more than a few, but none more shocking than when we went in for my wife's twenty-week ultrasound.

I remember the scene quite vividly. It was late afternoon, and we had the small ultrasonography room to ourselves. Our two-year-old daughter was wandering around in her cute, curious way. It was just us and the technologist, a woman with short hair and a slight Russian accent. We told her that we didn't want to know the sex; we wanted to be surprised.

She worked quietly for a few minutes. "Maybe you'll get one of each," she said at last.

My wife furrowed her brow and looked from her to our daughter. "Well, I guess if we had a boy, sure, we'd have one of each."

"No, one of each. It's twins, right?"

I'd been listening with half an ear—I'd long ago learned that in the maternity ward, husbands were regarded as furniture. But that last line caught my attention.

"What?" I asked.

"It's twins," she repeated.

My wife shook her head. This was the *twenty-week ultrasound*. There had to be some mistake. I didn't believe it until I marched over to the ultrasound machine and heard the two separate infant heartbeats. The realization left us in stunned silence. What are the odds, right?

I had a pretty fair idea of the odds, actually, because I happen to be a genetics researcher. Twins have long been valued by the research community because they're built-in genetics experiments. The incidence for twin pregnancies in the United States is about 33 per 1,000 births, or 3.3 percent.[*] The twinning rate has increased about 75 percent since 1980, primarily due to the rise of in vitro fertilization (which sometimes results in multiples). That didn't apply to our situation, nor did we have any family history. That made the odds of this happening about 2 percent.

Talk about a game changer. Our calm self-assurance evaporated faster than the last bottle of formula. We wouldn't have

---

[*] Centers for Disease Control, "Births: Final Data for 2018," *National Vital Statistics Report* 68, 13 (November 27, 2019), https://www.cdc.gov/nchs/data/nvsr/nvsr68/nvsr68_13-508.pdf.

the comfort of one-on-one coverage. With three kids and two grown-ups, we'd be playing zone defense at best.

Most of the baby gear we already had, the gear we'd counted on, came up short in the light of this unplanned doubling. We suddenly needed *another* car seat and *another* stroller and *another* crib. It was like starting over. On the bright side, we had time. We'd gotten the news later than usual, but this was only the twenty-week mark. We got to work with the renewed energy of first-time parents driven by a cocktail of excitement, fear, and uncertainty.

First things first, we needed a new vehicle. At the time, my wife drove a Honda CR-V. It was the perfect one-child car. Two children would have been doable. Three kids? No way. A twin stroller on its own is about the size of a small SUV. We visited a nearby car dealership to take a couple of large SUVs for a test drive. Somehow, even they didn't seem large enough. However, parked next to one of those insufficient SUVs was another type of vehicle. A vehicle that most people in my generation despised above all others. A vehicle that I'd sworn, at age seventeen, never to buy for myself.

A minivan.

This solemn vow is common among people my age who learned to drive their parents' first-generation minivan. The early models were built like tanks and carried immense social stigma when you were learning to drive. Or worse, when you had your license but access to no other car. Painful as they were, those memories faded away when my wife and I looked inside the minivan on the lot. All I heard was angelic harp music. All I thought was *look at the cargo room.*

We bought the minivan and it was one thing down, a hundred to go.

/

About 10 percent of infants in the United States are born pre-term; that's an alarming incidence given all of the medical and emotional complications of premature birth. Many factors increase the risk of preterm birth. Preterm birth rates are higher, for example, for Black and Hispanic parents (13.6 percent and 9.4 percent) than for white and Asian parents (9.0 percent and 8.7 percent). Certain medical conditions, such as diabetes, can increase the risk of delivering early. Being underweight or over-weight before pregnancy is also a risk factor.

All that being said, the March of Dimes recognizes three major risk factors for preterm labor. The first risk factor is a history of delivering preterm—either a personal history or a family history. In other words, if you already delivered a pre-term baby or were born early yourself, you carry increased risk. There is undoubtedly an inherited component to this factor, but it remains poorly understood. The second major risk factor is a history of problems with your uterus or cervix. About 3 percent of women are born with a defect in the size, shape, or structure of the uterus. Cervical insufficiency—a condition in which a woman's cervix dilates too early during pregnancy—affects an estimated 0.5 percent of parents.

The third major risk factor for delivering early is being preg-nant with multiples.* The majority of twins (60 percent) and nearly all higher-order multiples (97 percent) are born before thirty-seven weeks' gestation. Early preterm birth—before thirty-four weeks—is very serious, and almost 20 percent of twins are born that early. In approximately one-third of cases, multiples are delivered early for medical reasons. But for most multiple preemies, it's not clear *why* they come early, only that they do.

---

* "Preterm Labor and Premature Birth: Are You at Risk?" March of Dimes, accessed April 14, 2020, https://www. marchofdimes.org/complications/preterm-labor-and-premature-birth-are-you-at-risk.aspx.

In other words, maybe my wife and I should have seen it coming.

At thirty-three weeks into the pregnancy, we got another surprise. It was around 11:30 on a Monday evening. We were settling down, watching a TV show before bed, both of us already in pajamas. My wife was enjoying her nightly cookies and milk—a late-night snack had become a must early into pregnancy—when she sneezed. And her water broke. Now, over the previous weeks there had been times when she thought her water broke. False alarms. When it really happened, there was absolutely no doubt.

The twins were coming, and they were coming *early*.

The next twelve hours were harrowing. We went right to the hospital, where my wife's parents met us to take charge of our two-year-old. My wife was quickly admitted and fussed over by the attentive nurses. They ignored me, as was customary. I tried to stay out of the way. By the middle of the night, things had calmed down somewhat aside from the contractions that had started on the way to the hospital. The nurses had left us alone in a dim, quiet room. Naturally, I thought it was a good time to catch some shut-eye. My wife quickly disabused me of this notion.

Instead I was roused to summon the nurses, who summoned the doctor, who agreed that it was time. We'd already decided on a c-section because there were two babies, but their early arrival made it a certainty. They made ready to wheel my wife into surgery.

At this point, to my surprise and discomfort, I found *myself* the subject of sudden scrutiny.

"Has the dad eaten anything tonight?" the doctor asked.

"I don't know," a nurse answered.

"We don't want him passing out on the floor."

"You don't have to worry about me," I assured them. "I'm a rock."

All of them burst out laughing.

"Have you ever heard a more classic answer?" the doctor asked her colleague.

They were still chuckling as they pressed more graham crackers on me and took us to the operating room.

Delivery went mercifully well. We became the proud parents of two baby boys. At thirty-three weeks' gestation, they were destined for a long stay at the neonatal intensive care unit. The NICU. It's a familiar place for parents of preemies. Ours was, simply put, amazing. The entire unit had been remodeled a few months before. There were private rooms, and our twins merited one of the larger ones.

Grandma and Grandpa came to visit with our two-year-old, who'd managed to keep them awake all night long. They were dragging and so was I, but we had a good visit. Some time later, with a team of wonderfully capable medical personnel handling the baby care, I finally caught that nap I'd wanted.

We spent a couple of months in the NICU. They were a blessing in many ways. My wife and I got to practice caring for twins with backup from an entire team of professionals. The boys were so *tiny*. About four pounds each. It turns out they do make diapers for preemies that small. They're about the size of a gum wrapper, or at least they seemed that way when I was trying to change them. One of the many benefits of the NICU is that they get the babies on a schedule. The boys ate one right after the other, and then slept. Of course, this also meant that our "off time" was reduced by half an hour at each end. But we soldiered on. The twins grew, and before I knew it, we were talking about going home.

Leaving the NICU is a fraught experience. You're so excited to be going home, but simultaneously terrified of being on your own. We liked having our support team, even if they were completely unimpressed with my swaddling skills. There was also an incredibly stressful car seat test. The idea is to ensure that the babies are strong enough to breathe while in a car seat. I had to lug both car seats in and put the boys into them, a process made far more difficult because they were still hooked up to all of the NICU monitors. Strapping a five-pound baby into a brand-new car seat is tricky; I don't care who you are. And when I'd done it, I had to stand back and watch the oxygen saturation levels along with the staff. If the levels dropped, we weren't going home that day. Even worse, if only one boy passed, he would be discharged while the other stayed. (Talk about separation anxiety.)

It's a good thing that *my* vital signs weren't being monitored. I'm sure my blood pressure shot well into the range of clinical hypertension. It was dicey, but the boys passed. Barely. We said our tearful goodbyes to the nurses. I drove all of us home. Then we realized the stark numerical reality: the kids in the Koboldt household finally outnumbered the grown-ups.

Of course, we were not entirely alone. Because the twins were preemies, we were issued portable life monitors that constantly measured their breathing, heart rate, and oxygen levels. The machines were about the size of a lunch box but weighed several pounds each. Long insulated wires ran from these to a pair of adhesive sensor pads that rested on each baby's torso. Though tedious and heavy to lug around, the life monitors reassured us that our preemies were all right. Otherwise I'm not sure we'd have slept ourselves. If a baby seemed to stop breathing, the alarms blared at ear-piercing decibels.

It turns out, this was a deliberate design feature of the monitors. The loud, jarring noise tends to jolt an apneic infant to take a deep breath. To gasp, in other words. Usually, in the next room, his parents were doing the same. Every time it happened, my exhausted mind first thought it was a tornado siren. Or an air raid alarm, even though we weren't at war. I'd stumble into the semi-dark room, find the sensor pad that had come loose, and reattach it. It was almost always a false positive. Usually one of the boys had pulled a sensor loose. Despite their comforts, I was glad to give those monitors back to the medical-equipment rental company. We were lucky because the cost of their month-and-a-half rental was mostly covered by our insurance. We were also lucky that they were durable and well-made, because they got banged around quite a bit. I later learned that the cost to buy just one monitor was more than we'd paid for the minivan. Yikes.

An eerie silence fell over the household after we exited the life-monitor phase. When the machines were gone, it was *just us*. Three kids under the age of three, and two sleep-deprived adults who were entirely responsible for their survival. The silence, of course, did not last long. There were two tiny, hungry mouths to feed and so many diapers to change. Oh, the diapers. They start out little and cute, don't they? Then you hit that milestone of solid food, and suddenly things get *real*. Even with the wondrous invention known as the Diaper Genie, you never quite control the smell of your home again.

I don't remember much from those first few months at home. That's mostly due to the sleep deprivation. Preemies seem to have shorter cycles of sleeping and eating, so there was always something to do. We were blessed that Twin B, the surprise guest at twenty weeks, played the role of the beta well. He can sleep through almost anything. His older-by-one-minute brother preferred to establish a role of sleeping light and getting up early. He and I spent many early mornings together, him with a bottle and me with my coffee. Side note: it was during this period that I went from casual pod coffee drinker to committed family-size carafe coffee drinker. I had my reasons.

Like many preemies, our twins have always been a bit on the small size for their age. I'm told this may continue for a while. We were blessedly spared any serious medical consequences, and for that I'm grateful. Twins have an unusual bond, and while they didn't develop their own language as some twins do, they quickly learned to collude against us. I remember quite clearly the day that they figured out how to operate the lever-style doorknobs in our house. It reminded me of that terrifying scene from Jurassic Park. *They're smarter than we realized, and they can open doors.* Our saving grace is their precocious older sister, who helps us keep them in line. Still, they all play together and get along remarkably well (for siblings, at least). In fact, maybe I should be more concerned. If the boys bring her over to their side, we'll truly be outnumbered.

The Other Side

BY SARA COHEN

All of my life, I was certain I wanted to be two things: a mother and a nurse.

In grade school, I had baby dolls that I dressed in real baby clothes. I would page through my mom's department-store catalogs because there was an entire section devoted to baby items. I remember looking at pictures of nurseries and using a Sharpie to circle the furniture and bedding I liked the most. Along with my plans for being a mom, I also knew I wanted to be a nurse who cared for sick babies. It was no surprise to anyone when I went to nursing school and started working in a pediatric intensive care unit immediately after graduation.

When my husband and I decided to start a family, I was working as a staff nurse in a neonatal ICU in Philadelphia. I loved my job. I loved my coworkers. Most importantly, though, I loved my patients and their families. I was working the job of my dreams, responsible for helping the smallest and most vulnerable patients not only live but thrive. As their nurse, I protected my patients from infection, encouraged their growth, comforted them when their families were not there, taught their parents how to care for them, and was able to discharge them home. Not every outcome was joyous, but I treasured my role in the lives of these little humans.

But it wasn't until I was twenty-nine weeks pregnant with my first son that I began to understand the fear and uncertainty born alongside a premature baby.

I walked to work like any other day, and aside from feeling a little off, I was ready to tackle the twelve-hour shift ahead of me. Partway through my shift, though, I was still feeling strange. I went to the floor above me to be checked by the labor and delivery staff. They put me on a fetal monitor, strapping blue and pink bands around my belly, and it showed that I was having regular contractions. That couldn't be; I wasn't feeling contractions. I was certain the monitor was wrong. A doctor I knew came in to check me, and her pleasant conversation stopped abruptly after she began her examination. She stood up quickly, and I knew something was wrong. I was four centimeters dilated, she said, and the baby was going to arrive soon if they did not intervene. Amid the shock of the news, a small voice whispered in my mind: *How did you not know this was happening?* It was my own body, but I felt nothing. I was a nurse, but I couldn't see the signs.

The rest of that time was a terrifying blur. The doctor called for more help. Several nurses ran in and I gave permission for them to try to stop the labor. I was given a shot in my arm of betamethasone, a steroid that helps mature the baby's lungs. The goal is to deliver two doses, twenty-four hours apart, to have the greatest benefits for the baby. The steroid may also reduce the chance of bleeding in the brain and prevent an intestinal infection called necrotizing enterocolitis (NEC), both devastating potential consequences of being born prematurely. My hospital bed was also adjusted so that my legs were higher than my head, to help reduce pressure from the weight of the baby on my cervix. At the same time, two IVs threaded into my arms started pumping hydration fluids and a medication called magnesium sulfate to help stop labor and protect the baby's brain. The goal was to slow contractions and hold off the delivery for as long as possible. I remember the nurses telling me everything they were doing, the names of the medications, the reason for positioning my bed the way they did, but I didn't hear them. I couldn't process it, not then. There were only two thoughts in my mind: my baby could not be born this soon, and I was willing to do anything to give him more time to grow and mature in my body.

A neonatologist I work with regularly came in to talk to me

about the implications of having a baby boy at twenty-nine weeks. Everything was explained to me as if I were a NICU nurse who was also about to give birth to a preemie. I imagine they were trying to respect my knowledge and experience, but every bit of my brain that should have been able to comprehend what was happening had somehow vanished. I was not a NICU nurse in that moment. I was a mother in premature labor, and I was terrified. At some point, I stopped being able to hear them talking to me, and I could only hear that voice in my head. *How could I not know I was in preterm labor?*

This was the day when being blissfully pregnant ended for me. Even though my pregnancy lasted—thankfully, mercifully—another five weeks, this was the day I started blaming myself for not being able to keep my baby safe in my body. I was in the hospital's antepartum unit, on bed rest, for almost two weeks. The contractions stopped with the help of the magnesium sulfate, or mag, but as soon as they would stop the infusion and start letting me out of bed, the contractions would start again. Mag is a miserable medication to take, and I cried every time they started it again. It made me feel extremely hot, and I was not allowed to eat solid foods, only clear liquids. It also made my brain fuzzy and I struggled to hold conversations. But eventually, I was allowed to go home and spent another three weeks there on bed rest.

Charlie was born at thirty-four weeks and one day. He was big for a preemie, weighing six pounds, ten ounces, and he had a ton of hair. But he also had a hard time breathing. I was able to hold him for a short time after he was born, but he was quickly taken to the NICU—the NICU where I work—for respiratory distress and grunting while breathing. My coworkers were now taking care of him. There was some comfort in knowing the doctors and nurses now attending to him, but I was angry I could not have him with me. Always a mother first.

When Charlie left me in the delivery room, he was breathing on his own, although I knew he was struggling. When I went to see him five hours later, after settling into my inpatient room and getting some rest, he was on a ventilator. New anger flared within me. I was angry that no one had called to tell me that he was *this* sick. I was resting just two floors above while my baby was intubated and put on a ventilator, and no one had even told me. I should have been there with him.

And when I was with him, I couldn't stay for long. Eventually, I had to return to my hospital room to rest and start pumping breast milk for Charlie. Sleep seemed impossible, knowing that my baby lay in a plastic box with tubes and wires and alarms. The nurses implored me to rest while I was in the hospital and not to spend too much time sitting at his bedside. I knew these words well; I'd recited them to countless parents before—before everything around me changed, before my familiar workplace morphed into an alien and deeply distressing world. Now, hearing these words made me angry. I can see now that my anger was not because of the words and actions of the staff, the people I worked with side by side as a nurse. But in those first days as Charlie's mom, I was afraid and deeply saddened. Was my baby in pain? Was he lonely when I left him to sleep in my hospital room? Was his premature birth, and therefore the tests and treatments he needed, my fault? My body should have been able to carry him for forty weeks. What had I done wrong? What had I not done enough of? At the root of these questions and frustrations was the sense that I had failed Charlie. These feelings manifested in anger at anyone who reminded me to get some rest, eat some food, and take care of myself.

Two days after delivering Charlie, I was discharged home with no baby to bring with me. I sobbed the whole way home. I felt like I was abandoning him.

The first time I called the unit to check on my son, I asked for Charlie's nurse. "Who? I don't know who Charlie is." Oh, right, I needed to ask for "baby Cohen's nurse." I complained to my husband for at least twenty minutes about that exchange.

He was not baby Cohen; he was Charlie. He was our son. He had a name. Why couldn't they use it?

Every day I saw him, there were new bruises on him where intravenous lines had been attempted. The heels of his poor feet had bandages all over them, every day, from blood work that was drawn. His cheeks were raw from the tape used to secure first his breathing tube, then his nasal cannula, and then his feeding tube. I wanted to know the story behind each mark on his body. I felt terrible that I wasn't there all of the time to comfort him through each procedure. I'd done all of these procedures hundreds of times myself, on other babies, but everything changed when it was my own child. Even though I trusted my colleagues to provide good care for my son, I couldn't ignore that most primordial instinct to hold and protect him myself.

Every tiny incursion into his body, every technical term spoken over my head, felt jarring as a parent. Had I made other parents feel the same way when I was caring for their babies? Was I being too sensitive now, or did I really have so limited an idea of how hard it was having a premature baby in the NICU? I started to pay attention to everything that made me feel extra emotion—every experience that made Charlie's stay just a little bit harder on me as a parent. I vowed that after this was over, I would return to work more empathetic and better informed.

Halfway through his stay in the NICU, I had a meltdown in the hallway. One of the neonatologists had seen me standing there and casually asked how I was doing. I responded by bursting into tears and telling her how guilty I felt for my son's early delivery. This sweet doctor who had worked side by side with me for many nights hugged me, but then she assured me that none of this was my fault and that I "knew better" than to feel responsible for it. She was just trying to help, but she didn't understand what I needed. I had reassured countless moms, some many times over, this same way: telling them they were not at fault for their baby's early entrance into the world. It occurred to me that all the times I had told moms they were "silly" for thinking they did anything wrong, or how "ridiculous" it was that they felt guilty, it was probably the least helpful thing I could have been doing. What did I need in that moment? I needed a hug, yes. I also needed someone to let me talk and cry about how I felt without telling me to stop feeling that way, or telling me that it was wrong to think it.

/

One day, close to the time when Charlie was scheduled to be discharged, I was walking into the unit to visit him when I heard a nurse yell across the NICU to his primary nurse, who had just come back from break, that "baby Cohen had a brady that needed stim."

Wait, what?

First of all, *his name is Charlie.* He is not baby Cohen; his name is Charlie. Second, a bradycardia with stimulation? This means that my baby's heart rate slowed down significantly, and the nurse had to intervene. Sometimes the intervention is as simple as a tap on the baby's foot or a slight repositioning of the head. Other times, the nose and mouth need to be suctioned, or the baby is given breaths with a bag and mask. This is a common occurrence in preemies, and something I counseled other parents through. As a nurse, the pathophysiology—the way different parts of a body work (or don't work) together—makes complete sense to me. As a mom, however, I wanted answers. Why did this happen? How low was his heart rate? When did he start having bradys? What level of intervention did he need? Also, this isn't something you just casually yell across the nursery. I can't overhear this information secondhand; I need to be told about it, have the circumstances explained.

The neonatologist came to talk to me and told me something along the lines of, "It's no big deal; all preemies do this at some point, especially wimpy white boys; you know this from working here, we see this all the time, it's really no big deal." I couldn't believe how upset I was. But more than that, I couldn't believe I was being told that my son's heart rate dropping was no big deal and that I shouldn't worry about it. That was the day I felt most like I was losing my mind—and could even lose my job if I didn't keep myself together.

I'd had a version of this same conversation with so many parents prior to my son's birth. We used the phrase "wimpy white boy" as a term of endearment for the Caucasian preemie boys who tend to need some extra help compared to girls and infants of color. It had never occurred to me that I could be offending a parent by describing their child this way, but it made me very upset. *His name is Charlie and the only thing I want you to call him is Charlie.*

I had also told countless parents that their child's heart rate dropping was no big deal and that most preemies experience it. I would say that because we see it in the NICU all the time, we know how to correct it, we know what usually causes it, and we see most babies outgrow it. But as a parent, hearing that your child's heart is beating in any way other than normal is deeply distressing, even for a seasoned professional like myself. It is a big deal, and no parent should be told not to worry about it. Boy, was I learning some lessons on the other side of these interactions.

One night, shortly after the brady situation, I spilled an entire bottle of my pumped breast milk in the middle of the night. I had just started pumping enough milk at one time that I could measure it in multiple ounces. I thought I put the lid on the bottle, but when I sleepily bumped into it, the lid was most certainly not in place. It tipped over, the milk spilled everywhere, and I yelled and then started crying. My husband woke up and thought something had happened to Charlie when he heard how upset I was. He was relieved that the baby was fine and reassured me that I would just make more milk next time I pumped. I vividly remember the exhaustion and frustration I felt in this moment. I can see now that my husband was trying to make me feel better. I also knew that there was no possible way he could comprehend the myriad emotions I was carrying. In that moment, however, I unloaded all of that sadness and fear, and my crying turned to sobbing—the kind where you can't catch your breath. I am pretty sure my husband still thinks this was all over spilled milk, but it was so much more than that.

I'd never been able to understand, before, why NICU moms were so fixated on how much milk they had left for their baby and so devastated whenever they spilled milk or accidentally left it out instead of refrigerating it. Pumping milk for my son was the one thing I could do for him when he wasn't with me. Other people could take care of him at the hospital, but I was the only one who could supply him with breast milk, and that mattered to me. Pumping milk for him helped me feel connected to him when I wasn't sitting at his bedside and helped alleviate some of the guilt I had for not being able to hold onto him for the full forty weeks.

/

Charlie was discharged from the NICU after two weeks. As a NICU nurse, I routinely took care of babies who stayed in our unit for months, which makes two weeks sound like no time at all. Being on the other side, though—being the mom—it felt like an eternity. Any amount of time that a parent is without their baby is too long.

Charlie came home, and I was so relieved to feel whole again.

But my story about preemies doesn't end here. My second son, Aaron, was also born prematurely after a very scary and challenging pregnancy. He was born by emergency c-section at thirty-four weeks and one day, exactly the same as his brother, just a few years later. I was not surprised by Aaron's premature birth, and I felt more prepared to navigate the NICU as a parent. Even so, our experience was challenging in new ways. Aaron spent almost a month in the NICU, the same unit where I still worked as a nurse, and his time there was harder than Charlie's. Aaron struggled to gain and maintain weight. He had brady episodes that continued for weeks and, when he was finally sent home, we had to keep him on an apnea monitor. He was not able to breastfeed because of a weak suck and low muscle tone, but he screamed when he was fed by bottle. I also seemed incapable of making breast milk for him. I decided to stop pumping for Aaron when he was around two months old. I was barely making an ounce at a time, despite taking medications and trying everything I could to increase my supply, and he required formula supplementation for extra calories. Taking pumping out of my day gave me a little more time to spend with Charlie, who was three years old and full of energy, and it was one less task for me to worry about. I felt like I was giving up, and the subsequent guilt was intense. It was the right thing to do, but it took years for me to allow myself to realize that.

When I was pregnant with Aaron, we decided he would be our last child, given the pregnancy complications, the miscarriage I had between the pregnancies with Charlie and Aaron, and concerns for future attempts. After Aaron was born, I felt a new wave of sadness and grief for never having a "normal" pregnancy or delivery. My babies never stayed in my hospital room with me. They did not come home with me when I was discharged. When I look at pictures from their first weeks, they're covered in wires and tubes. This grief goes beyond the feelings that my body failed me, or that I failed my children by not carrying them to forty weeks. It manifests itself in feelings of jealousy, and even anger, at times when I should feel nothing but joy: a friend or family member delivers a full-term healthy baby, is able to exercise up until the day they deliver, comments on having too much breastmilk and not enough room to store it, their baby eats well and gains weight—any and all of these things trigger my sense of grief and leave me feeling jealous and angry. The passage of time helps, seeing my kids grow and mature helps, talking to others who understand how this feels helps. Grief is still there, but it has subsided in severity.

Having an intimate knowledge of how I felt after delivering my own preemies greatly influenced the care I gave to parents when I went back to work in the NICU. I understood the emotions and the trauma that can accompany giving birth prematurely, and I recognized that these feelings don't end when the baby is discharged from the NICU. I listened to parents, encouraged them to talk about how they felt, and urged them to continue talking to people once their baby came home. I have kept in touch with several of the parents whose babies I cared for in the NICU over the years. We bonded because I took care of their babies, but even more than that, because I was a preemie mom who understood them.

Charlie is now fourteen years old and Aaron is eleven. They are big, healthy boys, and I have had a lot of time to heal, but I will never forget what their early arrival taught me about myself—as a mother and as a NICU nurse.

Monstrous

BY ANNE THÉRIAULT

Every birth story makes sense only in retrospect. You spend months planning for the event, even though you know it's not really possible to plan. You collect other people's stories and try to see yourself in them: what you would do the same, what you would do differently. It gives you a sense of control. Afterward, once the baby is here, once they have finally come ashore from that perilous journey, you try to piece it together into some kind of coherent narrative. The birth itself exists in the space between what you envisioned and the story you will someday tell; it is outside of time or else it is too much inside of time, unending rushes of pain, terror, joy. During birth, you transcend the body and you are nothing but the body, all at the same time.

Nothing about my son's arrival went the way I'd expected. In fact, nothingness was the first sign that he was on his way: at thirty-four weeks' gestation, I suddenly stopped feeling him move. After none of the usual get-your-baby-moving tricks worked, I took the bus to the hospital, praying the whole way there for a stray kick or poke. No such luck. Once I arrived, I was whisked up to the maternity ward, where they hooked me up to an array of monitors and listened for a heartbeat. I'd been trying not to panic up until then, but the Doppler was eerily silent.

"He's dead," I wailed. "He's dead, I know he's dead."

Then the nurse moved the probe to the other side of my belly and there it was: the galloping sound of his tiny heart.

That first crisis resolved, the nurse turned to look at the readings on one of the machines I was hooked up to.

"Do you know you're having contractions?" she asked.

I said no, not that I could feel.

"That's strange," she said. "They're pretty strong."

Someone did a cervical check on me and said that I was two centimeters dilated, but not to worry: it was common to be a few centimeters dilated for days or even weeks before giving birth. Someone else wheeled in an ultrasound machine and, after a few passes of the wand, asked me if I knew that my baby was breech—feet first, in fact. I hadn't known that, either.

After an hour or so, the nurse did another cervical check and told me that I was five centimeters dilated. The contractions were still happening, according to the readout on the monitor, although I still couldn't feel them. In the rapid-fire way that some medical people have, the nurse told me three things that I had to come to terms with almost immediately: I was in labor, I would be having a c-section, and I wouldn't be going home until the baby was born.

The obstetrician on call wanted to do the surgery that night, saying that my membranes were close to rupturing—my water was going to break—and the baby's position put him at a high risk for an umbilical cord prolapse. I hadn't even thought about having a c-section, let alone a preterm c-section, besides knowing that I didn't want one. Instead, I'd pictured myself having a drug-free birth, the kind where you listen to Enya and bounce on a yoga ball and channel your inner goddess; the closest I'd gotten to thinking about interventions had been coaching my partner to remind me why I didn't want an epidural even if in the moment I really, really thought I wanted one. I remembered wishing a few days earlier that my pregnancy wouldn't go past forty weeks. I pictured one finger closing on the monkey's paw: let's grant her this and see how she likes it.

While I was stewing in my guilt—about my wish, as well as a vaguer guilt about not carrying the pregnancy to term—two patients needing emergency c-sections came through the ward. By the time an operating room was available for me, my contractions had stopped. I begged the obstetrician to hold off on the surgery, and he agreed on the condition that I be admitted to the hospital because it wasn't safe for me to go home. They would, he said, do the c-section either when my contractions started again or when I reached full term.

As it turned out, I had the surgery before either scenario could happen. After a week and a half on bed rest at the hospital, my obstetrician—a kindly older man who visited me every morning before his office hours began—told me that with every day that went by, I was making them more and more nervous that my water would break and the baby would be injured. I relented, and I was wheeled into the operating room the day I hit thirty-six weeks.

The surgery wasn't as bad as I'd thought it would be. At the very least, it was over quickly. There's something to be said for a planned c-section—at least I had time to prepare for it mentally. What I wasn't prepared for was my obstetrician turning to someone else present at the operating table (intern? resident?) and saying, "Ah, here's the reason the baby is breech." I had the odd sense of being object, not subject: a body on a table being discussed without being invited to participate in the discussion. But also, I was desperately curious to know what he meant.

I chimed in and somebody—I think my obstetrician—said that my uterus was bicornuate. Split into two chambers, like a cat's. A secret tucked up inside of me, invisible even on the ultrasounds I'd had. This shape limited my son's movements; he wasn't able to shift and turn head-down for delivery. Later, once my son had been extracted and weighed and wrapped up in a flannel blanket, I asked again about my uterus. How had it caused a breech birth? The nurse, who was busy doing something with all of the tubes coming out of my arm, said in an offhand way that it explained a lot, actually. A septum—a muscular band of tissue—split it in two, which meant that my son had run out of room, which was probably why I'd gone into labor early. It could also, she said, cause growth restrictions, which might be why even at thirty-six weeks he was still only just over five pounds.

My son and I were wheeled over to the recovery room, where I hoped we'd have some time to bond, but after a few minutes there another doctor was called to monitor the baby's breathing. He was grunting, they said, which wasn't good. They packed him up in a little bassinet and wheeled him away, my husband trailing behind. My mother was off somewhere calling everyone she could think of to announce that she was a grandmother. I was left alone, unable to move; I felt like a piece of land that had been excavated, stripped of everything valuable and then abandoned. A nurse came over to show me how to express colostrum, which apparently meant that she was going to squeeze my breasts painfully until it came out. Except the liquid that came out was brownish-red instead of the usual golden color. The nurse shook her head and said it was rusty pipe syndrome, something that happens when blood leaks into your milk ducts. She reassured me that it would still be fine to breastfeed, but all I could think was *Jesus, can't my body do anything right?*

How long was my son gone for? My concept of time kept expanding and dwindling, so I'm not sure. Long enough for them to feed him sugar-water because I wasn't there to try to nurse. Long enough for them to move me out of recovery and into a room on the maternity ward. Long enough for me to look up what a bicornuate uterus actually is. As it turned out, there were other possible complications that the nurse hadn't mentioned: increased incidence of miscarriage, fetal abnormalities, and placental problems, to name a few.

Up until everything went sideways, my pregnancy had been physically easy but mentally harrowing. I'd developed a paranoia that anything and everything could hurt the baby: people bumping into me on the subway, the two glasses of beer I'd had before I found out I was pregnant, the possibility of contaminated food. I worried about lead paint on our walls and *listeria* in deli sandwiches. For months, I'd been carrying around a tattered list of fish ranked according to their average mercury content so I knew what was safe to eat if I was at a party or a restaurant. A few weeks before I went into labor, when I knew my anxiety was out of control but had no idea how to stop it, I had a meltdown about red wine vinegar: what if it gave the baby fetal alcohol syndrome? I knew that it couldn't, but I had an equal sense that I didn't know what was real anymore. All I could be sure of was that the world was full of danger, and the baby was at risk. Then, when I was sitting alone in my hospital bed scrolling through articles about uterine malformations, I knew with a terrible clarity that all along my body itself had been the biggest threat.

All those long months of my pregnancy, I'd tried to convince myself that I was overthinking things, that my fears were unfounded, that I was being unreasonable. Now I wondered if it had been intuition—the skill that's supposed to be gifted to mothers magically—telling me that something was wrong. Because something *had* been wrong. I'd been right about that, even if I hadn't been looking in the right direction. That thought was strangely validating in the middle of my creeping terror, but it didn't erase the fact that what had failed was my body. I felt monstrous when I thought of my body growing new life at the same time that it was endangering that life. My body, I suddenly realized, was wildly untrustworthy, and as a consequence I felt untrustworthy as a mother; if my uterus could hurt my baby without me even knowing it, what other harm was I capable of?

Meanwhile, my son was still off in some other part of the hospital. First, he was on a continuous positive airway pressure (CPAP) machine to help with his labored breathing; then they trundled him through the underground tunnels to the adjoining children's hospital to do X-rays; then more CPAP. When they eventually brought him back to me, he had an IV port in his tiny hand for antibiotics. They had found fluid in his lungs, and they weren't sure if it was pneumonia or just retained amniotic fluid. His breathing was better but, the nurse cautioned me, still not perfect; he could stay with me for now, but he might have to go to the neonatal intensive care unit. They weren't sure yet. Meanwhile, I should try to feed him.

The feeding did not go well. I tried everything they'd taught us in our birthing class—make a hamburger with your nipple, hold the baby like a football, squish his open mouth onto the breast when he cries—but he just couldn't latch. That night, we fed him with a tube and a syringe, and then the next day I expressed more colostrum into a tiny medicine cup and we used that, but I still worried that he wasn't getting enough. I attended classes with a hospital lactation consultant, asked the nurses for help, patiently listened while my mother explained what latching was supposed to feel like, but ultimately no matter how helpful everyone was, they couldn't breastfeed for me. I would cry through each feeding, thinking: *my body is failing again, it is bad at this, I am bad at this, I am a bad mother.*

Fortunately, my son didn't have pneumonia, and he avoided a NICU stay. We were discharged a few days later, even though my son still wasn't eating or gaining weight properly. He was getting so few calories, he didn't have the energy to stay awake through feedings. The lactation consultant told me to undress him and tickle his feet and blow on his face to keep him alert and sucking; needless to say, nursing sessions turned into bigger productions and I started to dread them even more. I rented a pump from the hospital, but my son refused to take a bottle. My son also didn't sleep well, probably because he was constantly hungry. My mother tried to tell me that it was fine to quit breastfeeding, but I refused to listen. My body had already failed—I kept coming back to that word over and over—and I was not going to let it fail again. If I hadn't been producing enough milk, that would have been one thing; but the lactation consultant had assured me that my supply was abundant, and my son was clearly hungry. I hated myself more with every passing day; I couldn't do pregnancy right and now I couldn't even make sure my child was fed, arguably the most fundamental task of motherhood.

I became convinced that something was wrong with my son.

Something secret, invisible to the naked eye, like my cloven uterus. If it wasn't something I'd done, then it was something I was doing, something I didn't even know was bad; I had the sense once again of not knowing what reality was. I thought I heard him grunting again, like he had in the hospital. I thought maybe he wasn't getting enough oxygen. I thought maybe he had brain damage. Imagine: you bring a perfect baby into the world and then you hurt him without even realizing it. I knew that once the authorities got wind of it, they would take him from me, because I was clearly unfit.

I fantasized about dying, which I knew was another sign that I was a bad mother. Meanwhile, I was gamely posting social media updates about life as a new mom, and my friends and family would reply with comments that only made me feel worse: that I must be so happy, that I shouldn't sweat the small stuff, that I should enjoy these days while they lasted because someday I'd miss them. I couldn't sleep even though I was exhausted, and I would stay up late into the night, searching online for what might be wrong with my baby and crying over every result.

Eventually, after two months, there was a denouement. I broke down in front of someone, they made me go to the doctor, I started taking medication and was placed on a waiting list for a support group. The lactation clinic at the hospital gave me a nipple shield, and my son began gaining adequate weight and hitting milestones. I made friends with other parents of children around my son's age, and developed a better context for his development. By the time a spot opened up in the support group, I was already in a much better place, if only because watching my son hit milestones and seeing him around other babies had convinced me that he was fine. Nine years later, he still seems fine. I continue to have brief moments of paranoia—is he slower than his peers to master one skill or another because I ate too much fish when I was pregnant?—but mostly I'm okay. The dust has settled. I can tell his birth story confidently now because I know how it ends.

I don't really tell it thoroughly, though, unless I know my audience. My memories of my first two months of mother-hood—which, let's be honest, felt two decades long—are dark and chaotic. I hate that his entry into this world was so marred by my own fear. I'd wanted so badly for his birth to be joyful, and I still feel guilty admitting that it was mostly anything but. There must have been good moments. Didn't I cry with joy when he wailed for the first time? Didn't I look at his face with wonder and awe? But what I remember most is the disruption, the long hours I spent alone while he, separated from his mother, had to undergo tests and treatments. I am grateful that he's here and he's healthy, but I still grieve his birth. Did it have to be that way? Could any of it have been different? That's a dangerous path to go down, not to mention an unsatisfying one, because I'll just never know.

And sometimes I still wonder about that monstrous mother. What else lurks inside me that I don't know about? I don't neces-sarily mean physical hazards. I suppose I mean unmotherly ten-dencies, selfish desires, frustrations, fears; sometimes they come bursting out and I yell or cry or lock myself in the bedroom. What if I am not a good mother? Is there even such a thing as a good mother? When will I finally know? It's something else that, I suspect, will only make sense in retrospect.

New Year's Blessing

BY SHAWN SPRUCE

Late one summer evening, I returned home to Cherokee, North Carolina, from a business trip. Brooke, my partner, was waiting, slightly more upbeat than usual, although I didn't pick up on it at the time, and she handed me a small box wrapped in plain white paper. Expecting a simple gift, I opened it nonchalantly. Inside I found only a smooth white plastic stick laid neatly on a piece of cotton. Printed on one end were three purple letters: "EPT." It took me a moment to realize what it meant. I felt very happy, very proud, and very confident as I hugged and kissed Brooke and we began the next chapter in our lives together.

I had first traveled to Cherokee from New Mexico for work six years earlier, never imagining it would become my home. Much greener and more welcoming than the reserved Pueblo communities of my own people, I felt an instant connection to the land, the culture, and the people of western North Carolina. Then, two years later, I met Brooke at a meeting one evening in Snowbird, the community where her family is from, and my life changed completely—for the better, of course, as our whirlwind romance quickly evolved into more.

Brooke and I were now thrilled with our good news. We had been trying to conceive for nearly a year, and we had been growing impatient. But we agreed to keep quiet for a few months, happily keeping our shared secret from family and friends. We wanted it to be just about us for as long as possible, and we would plan a fun party later to make our announcement to the family. Our baby was due on March 8, so we thought we had plenty of time.

Two weeks later, I received an unexpected email from a retired nurse, back in Albuquerque, who had worked with my late father many years ago during his residency. A former colleague had sent her an old photo that she in turn forwarded to me. My dad died young, in his thirties, but I've always been especially proud of his career as an obstetrician.

The picture was one I had never seen before, taken while my dad was on call. He was wearing scrubs, a necktie, and a warm smile. I was awestruck by the serendipity, thinking to myself: *He knows. He knows, and he is happy.* A closer look at the image revealed a handsome young doctor leaning casually against a desk. Head tilted slightly, hands folded on his lap, the man exuded a calm confidence. It seemed almost as though he was reassuring me and Brooke that he would be there for our family, just as he had been there for his own family more than forty years before. Another fact I've always treasured: he delivered me when I was born.

Brooke has her own unusual birth story. She was born prematurely at twenty-eight weeks, and she weighed one pound, eleven ounces. I was reminded of this fact every November 17—World Prematurity Day—when Brooke made sure I wore something purple. But we never imagined history might repeat itself with our child.

We held out for as long as we could, but at fourteen weeks' gestation we invited Brooke's parents and two sisters to Sunday dinner. After the meal, I told them I wanted to show a video I had made during a pow wow we had all attended earlier that summer. They loved it. Watching the brightly outfitted fancy dancers swirl and a short clip of Brooke braiding the hair of her younger sister, Dakota; laughing at scenes of everyone hanging out, telling jokes. At the three-minute mark, Brooke's mother, Sandy, is seen relaxing on a lawn chair as the sun begins to set, pleasantly lamenting about not having grandchildren. She looks toward the camera and tells me how much fun it would be if Brooke and I had five children. I laugh nervously before telling her I'm going to have to get another job. Sandy looks disappointed but smiles, holds up a finger, and cheerfully pleads, "Oh, Shawn, then just start with one."

The video faded to black and a small bright image appeared, gradually expanding in size. By now, Brooke's bewildered family were all hunched over, staring intently at the screen. Finally, the image became clear: an ultrasound photo. Brooke's father, Diamond, spoke first in his hearty Eastern Cherokee drawl—"Baby"—followed by a brief moment of silence before Sandy cried out. Immediately, she and her daughters, Dakota and Wahlalah, began jumping wildly around the room, arms flailing, dancing and screaming in delight. Sandy hugged Diamond, now teary-eyed, and exclaimed, "Dad, we're going to be grandparents!" Meanwhile, the sisters continued their celebratory antics, while their two boyfriends looked on awkwardly. Brooke and I held hands from the side of the living room, marveling at how beautifully our plan came together and the joy we created.

/

Four months later, on New Year's Eve, I drove Brooke to the obstetrician a few miles away, in the town of Sylva, for a routine afternoon appointment. Along the way we made plans for a relaxing evening at home, watching the ball drop and snacking on popcorn. Little did we know what that New Year's Eve had in store for us.

A few weeks before, the doctor had warned that our pregnancy might not go full-term. It was nothing too alarming; just an issue with Brooke's blood pressure that might require inducing labor a few weeks early. But Brooke was being monitored closely, and her blood pressure seemed to be under control.

At the doctor's office, though, we learned that the situation had changed. Although she felt fine, Brooke's blood pressure had become dangerously elevated, creating a serious pregnancy complication known as preeclampsia. Left unchecked, the condition poses tremendous risks to mother and baby—possibly resulting in seizures, cerebral hemorrhage, even death.

Brooke was admitted to the regional hospital in Sylva for observation at 4:00 p.m. The doctors there explained that if they could get her blood pressure under control, she could probably go home the next morning. But after three hours of bed rest and medication, she hadn't improved. Brooke was transferred to a larger hospital an hour away in Asheville, which had the only neonatal intensive care unit in western North Carolina.

In Asheville, doctors again tried to curb Brooke's blood pressure, which had spiked even higher during the ambulance ride. At 11:30 p.m., with Brooke's blood pressure still soaring, we were told the baby needed to be delivered immediately via Cesarean section. By this time, Brooke's sisters had arrived from Cherokee. Brooke's parents were three states away on business, unable to make it home on such short notice but calling every few minutes for updates.

A team of medical staff descended upon us. They explained the procedure and its risks, and began preparing Brooke for surgery. I finally grasped the enormity of the situation and felt myself begin to shut down. Brooke noticed immediately and reached for my hand. "You need to be strong now, okay? For us, you need to be strong." I can best describe her tone as one of earnest compassion. A few minutes later, an anesthesia technician shook my hand and wished me a Happy New Year. I glanced at a clock on the wall; the time was 12:10 a.m. We were given a few minutes to pray as a family before Brooke was wheeled away to the delivery room. Because of the nature of the emergency, I was not allowed in the delivery room until the moment before the baby was born. A friendly nurse helped me into a surgical gown and led me to a small waiting room where I paced the floor and stared at my shoes for what felt like hours. I had done everything I could up to this point, and it was time now to put my trust in God and medicine.

We welcomed our beautiful daughter, Celeste Shawna Spruce, into the world at 1:12 a.m. on New Year's Day. We were blessed that the delivery went extremely well for both mother and baby. Born nine and a half weeks premature, our baby girl was "tiny but mighty," a nurse told me. Celeste tipped the scales at a whopping three pounds, three ounces, stretching sixteen inches from head to toe.

Many people had told me I would cry the first time I saw my newborn child. But I didn't. Not in the delivery room, not following the nurses who transferred our daughter to the neonatal intensive care unit, not later, watching her sleep safely in an isolette, a tangle of small wires and tubes keeping her fragile body alive. Seven hours later, nurses brought Brooke to the NICU to hold our baby for the first time. As I watched Brooke finally take our newborn daughter, squirming and sobbing, into her arms and tenderly kiss her delicate round nose, I felt a tear roll down my cheek.

That afternoon, reporters stopped by the hospital to interview the proud but exhausted parents of the New Year's Baby. Later, friends wrote us messages about how they'd seen our story on the evening news or read about it on the front page of the newspaper. The following morning, Brooke's parents met their first grandchild after driving eighteen hours through a vicious cold snap. They reminded us that Brooke had spent the first two and a half months of her life in the very same NICU as Celeste. Later, we even had the opportunity to meet one of the doctors who had cared for Brooke thirty years before. I decided to wear extra purple in November from then on.

The next few days and weeks were draped in a sense of solitude—stressful and tiring but sometimes oddly soothing—as the life I had known came to an abrupt halt. For the first eight days, time seemed to stand still; Brooke and I didn't even go outside. It was as though the entire world around us evaporated as our days and nights merged into countless trips back and forth between Brooke's hospital room and the NICU to help care for our precious young daughter. Our one indulgence came at 2:00 a.m. every morning, when the hospital cafeteria reopened for the graveyard shift and we stole away for ice cream bars.

I was grateful that my work was slow because of the holidays, and I didn't have any trips scheduled. I was shocked, sometimes, to remember the plans we had made for that time—the time we were supposed to be getting ready for our March baby, when instead we were learning how to care for a tiny human for six weeks in the hospital.

As a parent, you think you're prepared—you try your best to get ready—but you really have no idea what you're going to encounter until the day arrives. You also discover insecurities that you didn't know existed. When a baby is born, I found, dads can be overlooked while mothers are showered with attention and praise. Whether real or imagined, there were times I felt dismissed, underappreciated, and isolated. Being far away from my family and friends in New Mexico didn't help. For the first time, I understood how a younger, less mature, or less secure father might choose to leave. Not that I ever considered it or condone it, but now I better understand how it can happen. Sometimes, when I felt overwhelmed, I returned to that image on my phone of my own father. I felt closer to him than I had in years.

Thankfully, there was an extremely cool male nurse in the NICU—the only male nurse, in fact—named Andy. When I first met Andy, he didn't exactly fit the image in my mind of a NICU nurse. Broad and stocky with a reddish-brown beard and thick hands, he looked better suited to weld oil rigs than nurture delicate newborn babies. Looks can be deceiving. Because Brooke was still recovering from her surgery, I was the parent more often in the NICU during that first week. It was during this time that I gave Celeste the nickname I still call her by today, Munchie, because to me she looked like a little munchkin baby. Under Andy's guidance, I gave Munchie her first bath, learned to change a diaper, and shuttled bottles of breast milk to the NICU. Andy made me much more appreciative of my role as a father. I respected his knowledge and expertise, while his dry sense of humor helped put me at ease.

Andy also taught me the importance of holding and touching a preemie baby as often as possible, so the infant knows she is loved and protected. Once, as I stood with gloved hands gently resting on my daughter's back, Andy appeared by the bedside with a handful of paper squares and a bottle of black ink. While we made placards of Celeste's footprints, a tradition I remember from my own childhood, Andy held up one of my daughter's little ink-stained soles and quipped, "So I take it you must be a member of the Blackfeet tribe." I couldn't help but enjoy a good laugh.

/

When we finally came home in mid-February, real life kicked in quickly, with changing diapers, feeding the baby, going back to work, and all of the other tasks that move the days forward. It was only later that I began to realize how tremendously stressful and difficult those six weeks of Celeste's NICU stay had actually been. It's human nature, I believe, to block out emotionally traumatic experiences like these, and as our children grow we are constantly faced with new parenting challenges that pull us even further away from the beginning. Once we got back on our feet, I just wanted to move on.

Celeste celebrated her sixth birthday a few months ago. Looking at her now—when I drop her off at kindergarten on a cold morning, go swimming on a summer day, wrestle playfully on the living room floor, or take her with me on a business trip—it's hard to imagine she was once a frail little preemie who barely weighed three pounds or how our lives came to such a complete standstill that New Year's Day.

Every year on Celeste's birthday, however, Brooke returns to that time and place, delivering a gift basket full of baby products and treats to the family of the New Year's baby. Brooke has also become a prematurity awareness advocate, participating in the annual March for Babies walk, attending prematurity conferences, and volunteering on the NICU parent advisory council and as a parent-to-parent support provider at the hospital where she and Celeste were born.

A good friend had a baby recently. When I visited and reached out to hold the baby, I had to remind myself how to support a newborn's head and cradle her small body. Has it really been that long?

I'm awestruck, during this time that can seem both impossibly long and dizzyingly short, that my daughter and I are like passing ships as our lives briefly align for her ephemeral childhood. I've read that by the time a child graduates high school, she will have consumed 90 percent of the in-person time she will ever spend with her parents.

Every year also brings a new set of parenting challenges, and no parent is equally suited to handle the different responsibilities throughout every stage of a child's growth. So I don't believe there is such a thing as a great parent. Very good parents, yes. But no parent is great. Along with a photo of Michael Landon, who played Charles Ingalls, the ultimate TV dad from my childhood, there is a quote that hangs on my bathroom wall: "Like the attempt to make a work of art, being a father is an ongoing encounter between a man's ideal notion of himself and the sobering truth of his limitations. As they go about the precious work of creation, the best artists, like the best fathers, seem achingly aware of where they themselves fall short, still hoping all the while to realize their original conception."[*]

Brooke and I are raising our daughter, as best we can, to be

---

[*] Lee Siegel, *Wall Street Journal*, "A Portrait of the Artist as a Great Father" (June 15, 2018).

a strong woman who will represent herself and her people with dignity, wisdom, and character. Sometimes I like to think about the circle of love surrounding her—aunts, uncles, and grandparents—and how that circle extends above and below her. Celeste is now older than I was when my own father passed away, but she asks me about him sometimes, and I take comfort in telling her that he still watches over us.

The Still, Small Voice

BY KELSEY OSGOOD

I always associate disaster with loud noise or great activity: a skyscraper-sized wave crashing onto the beach, a nuclear reactor exploding with a deafening roar, a gun firing. It seems odd to have panicked, then, over the opposite: a slow fade, a quieting, some mysterious retreat.

Early in the morning of Wednesday, November 14—probably sometime between 2:00 and 3:00 a.m., though I no longer remember exactly when—I woke up to scratch myself. I was, by this point, thirty-four weeks and six days pregnant with my second child. The itching had started a few days prior: late one night earlier that week, I had gotten up to pee, and I noticed that my legs were tingling. The next night, I was clawing myself so hard in my sleep that my husband had to rouse me; in the morning, I had a crosshatch of blood on my distended stomach. He found me that night in the bathroom, rubbing the palms of my hands with my bristled hairbrush, and led me sadly back to bed, like I was a somnambulist who'd been caught perched on a windowsill.

It had been the latest in a string of horrors that I felt had marred my second pregnancy, a marked contrast from my carefree first. When my older child was a tiny zygote, he passed every test with flying colors, and I marched through the entire pregnancy with completely undeserved confidence and few discomforts, save some nasty heartburn in my third trimester. One of my most enduring memories of the forty weeks was once, sitting in the waiting room at the ultrasound facility, I was drinking ice-cold water from a tiny paper cone and surveying the *OK!* magazines fanned out on the table, and a massively hubristic thought popped into my head: *I don't even need to be here, because I know with 100 percent certainty that this baby is fine.* And he was.

This second time, however, was different. As before, I'd gotten pregnant quickly, just before my first son's first birthday, in March. The morning sickness was slightly more severe, but I'd heard that could be the case. The first blip came that summer when we were visiting my father's family in Michigan, and the secretary at my doctor's office called to give me the results of my blood test.

"He told you about the low PAPP-A?"

I told her I had no idea what she was talking about. She bumbled through an explanation—I sympathized with her lack of articulation, as of course she wasn't a doctor—and suggested having my obstetrician call me back. That afternoon, we drove up north to a lake, and I spent my time intermittently tossing toys back at my fourteen-month-old and frantically searching online. I found pages that said low PAPP-A—a hormone that ensures placental health—was associated with increased risk of stillbirth, preeclampsia, intrauterine growth restriction, and early delivery; I also found a number of studies that said the connection between low PAPP-A and any of those outcomes was tenuous at best. Eventually I fixated on a thread on some random pregnancy forum that was equal parts terrifying and reassuring: in a series of posts, parents unleashed their fears about their unborn children in grammatically dubious rants. The contributors covered everything from their low PAPP-A to the risks of Down syndrome and trisomy 13, a genetic condition that causes intellectual disability and physical defects—the connection between the two, if there is one, was unclear—but then wrote follow-ups informing readers that their anxiety had been for naught, because their babies were born healthy at term. "PLEASE do yourself a favor and don't google a damn thing again about pregnancy," one parent wrote, in what became a soothing refrain.

Of course, we know too much, and we worry too much! I thought.

When the afternoon dragged on and the doctor still hadn't called me back, my husband insisted we contact the on-call doctor from the practice. I spoke to her while pacing the parking lot of a rural Michigan road stop as tank trucks barreled by.

"How worried should I be?" I shouted into the phone.

"Not ... very." I could hear something in her voice: Was it boredom? "We see a lot of low PAPP-A and a lot of good outcomes. You'll probably just have to take a baby aspirin every day—although I think that advice has changed recently? You'll have to ask your doctor when you speak to him."

Over the ensuing months, I tried to maintain a casual pregnant lady persona, making endless jokes to friends about second pregnancies—how much less magical they were, laughing and pretending as though it was, by now, all so routine as to be almost dull. But underneath my blasé veneer, vague, dark fears lingered. In the sticky early days of summer, I'd drape myself exhaustedly on top of my bed, touch my rising belly, and think about how my mother's second pregnancy had been a miscarriage, so it would make sense if *my* second one was, too. My armor of confidence had been removed: I had already been touched by prenatal complications, so why not miscarriage? When the technician at my twenty-week growth scan congratulated me, I almost snapped that she was being presumptuous. And even if the fetus was fine now, I figured, that's because it just wasn't late enough in the pregnancy: low PAPP-A was associated with a decline in placental strength as the gestation progressed, so as my due date approached, that warm organ within which my baby slept could—in my mind, *would*—disintegrate and die. It was only a matter of time.

/

When I was pregnant with my first child, we were living in England. I frequently hung out with two close friends: Linnea, the wife of my friend from college, who had recently given birth to her first child, and Esther, a midwife who worked for a National Health Service hospital. Linnea had been induced two weeks before her due date because she had developed cholestasis, a liver functionality problem specific to pregnancy in which the bile acids in the blood build up and cause severe itching, specifically on the hands and feet but sometimes all over the body, among a few other symptoms like depression and dark urine. Women with cholestasis are often induced a few weeks early because the condition is correlated with an increased risk of stillbirth as the pregnancy continues.

"I used to go to the bathroom during work just so I could pull down my pants and scratch myself," Linnea told me once, over lunch. Shortly after she said this, I noticed that my own legs were itchy: when I took off my tights at the end of the day, I'd often scratch my thighs until they were just pink.

"Do you think I have cholestasis?" I asked Esther, who, by pure coincidence, happened to run a clinic for women with the condition.

She shrugged. "Maybe it's just that it's wintertime and your skin is dry? Is the itching *really* bad?" Never having been good at rating pain, I demurred. Shortly thereafter, I was diving down some Internet wormhole, and landed on an essay by the playwright Sarah Ruhl on her own experience with cholestasis. "This was no casual itch," she wrote. "I scratched until I bled. I applied lotion. I put on a humidifier. I scratched. I rubbed ice on my body." That sounded a lot more serious than slightly prickly thighs in January.

What are the odds of having a friend who had a rare condition, knowing a midwife who specializes in it, and randomly stumbling on an essay by someone who had it? Pretty slim, I figured. I must have psychosomatically created the itching. For a moment,

I giggled at how funny and powerful the mind was, then I vowed to forget about the itching, which I promptly did.

Fast forward nearly two years: I'd been basically unable to eat for weeks, as the result of severe heartburn. It was far worse than in my first pregnancy: one falafel sandwich made me so sick for an entire day that I had to sleep sitting bolt upright in bed. I felt like chunks of food were perpetually lodged in my throat. I was told not to eat or drink at the same time and not to lie down until twenty minutes after eating, and to take papaya enzymes and to chew gum—the end result of which was just me gnawing on Trident constantly and never eating or sleeping or drinking anything at all, because even water hurt. I stopped gaining weight. I developed patches of dry, flaky skin under my eyes; a rash that had once lingered underneath a ring my father had given me bloomed again, then cracked before the skin peeled off. My calves seized up in the middle of the night so violently that I lurched out of bed. I felt my mood dip into melancholy, but the skies were getting grayer and the air colder, so that was probably seasonal, I reasoned. My doctor moved my due date back a few days, based on the baby's measurements; when I wondered aloud if that meant something was wrong—gently, as I had always strived to be an easy patient, as if that would somehow ensure a healthy outcome—he said no, that's just how things were done, even though I hadn't ever heard of that happening to anyone else. I had the curious sensation that my stomach was softening, shrinking, even, and a more frightening sense that the baby was kicking less frequently and less forcefully.

"I think the baby's kicks are getting weaker," I told my friend, who worked as a birth doula.

"It could be that the baby has turned backward and is kicking toward your spine," she said. "I'm sure everything is fine!"

"I am just a little worried that the baby isn't moving as much," I told my obstetrician, my legs dangling off the exam table.

"Well, you're much more active than you were in your first pregnancy!"

"I don't feel the baby kick as much," I said to my husband, about ten times a day.

"I'm sure it's because you're just out moving all the time. Don't get so stressed about it. I don't want to use the 'h' word but you're being a little ..." He trailed off before he could say *hysterical*.

When the cholestasis symptoms started, I was positive that's what it was, but I still listened to my husband try to convince me otherwise for two days. *Dry skin in winter* was his line. I felt like someone with Morgellons, a medically unrecognized condition in which people often believe bugs are crawling under their skin and causing them to itch, but for which no insect-related cause has ever been found. By day three, even my husband had to concede that something seemed amiss. I video-called Esther in London. I told her the night before, when my tingling palms woke me up at two, I had simply given up and gotten out of bed to watch movies and scratch myself for three hours. What was I supposed to do, stare at the wall and try to ignore it? I watched her facial expression shift nearly imperceptibly into that of a medical professional trying to keep her patient calm.

"You'll be absolutely *fine*," she said in her beautiful lilting accent. "Just call your doctor and tell him to give you a blood test." I told her I had an appointment that Friday; she said it could wait until then. "It's not an emergency," she said. Even then, I wondered if I would actually follow through or if I would try to tell myself to ignore it, in the hopes that not making trouble would somehow karmically work in my favor and the whole issue would just disappear.

That night before I went to sleep, I was scrolling through the Instagram feed of a design blogger, who had been updating her account less often since getting pregnant with her second child. She'd had her baby, but only after she'd been diagnosed with cholestasis and admitted to the hospital for a c-section. I sat paralyzed in my chair, watching the little slides she posted pass by: this one urging me not to worry about looking paranoid, the next saying it's better to get checked out even if you're sure things are fine. "I had a sixth sense something was not right and I couldn't shake it," she wrote. The penultimate picture was of a perfect little baby sleeping on her belly. I immediately emailed my doctor and told him I thought I had cholestasis. He responded seven minutes later. "We'll do the blood test on Friday."

I woke up in the black early morning and nestled back into my predawn spot in the crook of the couch, hairbrush in one hand and fork in the other, and turned on a movie. At some point I started to wonder how long it had been since I'd felt the baby move: since I'd woken up? Earlier that evening? Had I felt the baby move at all that day? Esther had taught me that in these scenarios, I should drink some juice, lie on my left side, and wait. All we had in our fridge was some possibly rancid pineapple juice, and the thought of drinking something acidic with my heartburn made me want to vomit—I had to come to envision my blood was almost pure acid, threatening to bubble out of every orifice— but I took the heftiest gulp I could muster and laid down. *I am here. I am listening.* A few minutes later, I felt the tiniest flutter, like someone tinkling three keys *pianissimo.* Then nothing.

In the stillness, every neuron in my brain fired; every muscle tensed, poised for action. *Go go go go go now go now.* I used to joke with friends that every thought I had went through three layers of analysis—the thought, the thought about the thought, and the thought about the thought about the thought—so I was unaccustomed to such visceral terror. I ran up the stairs to my bedroom like a wild animal, screaming and sobbing, "The baby, the baby!"

/

On the way to the hospital, I could only manage two coherent thoughts: *The lights on the Brooklyn Bridge look particularly beautiful tonight,* followed by *This baby is dead, and I'm going to have to labor and deliver him.* Years earlier, a friend of mine had her water break early, spontaneously, in her sixteenth week of pregnancy, and she was forced to give birth to the fetus who would have been her first daughter. She sent out a mass email to alert her friends to the news: "I just wanted you all to know," she wrote, "so you aren't wondering what happened the next time you see/talk to me." *That's very smart,* I thought at the time. In the back of the taxi that morning, I composed a similar letter in my head.

I had stopped crying by the time my obstetrician intercepted me at the check-in desk and led me by the hand to a small bed in triage. He and an ultrasound technician zipped the flimsy cloth curtain closed to afford us some privacy, but I could still hear a woman in the very early, placid stages of labor across the room. The lighting was low, and it seemed either calming or ominous; I couldn't decide. The technician squeezed the familiar chilly gel onto my stomach and placed the transducer probe on top. A faint but distinct whooshing sound pulsed through the cordoned area.

"There's the heartbeat," the technician said.

My doctor smiled brightly. "Mishegoss!" he announced with glee, gathering up his papers. "They're going to keep you here for a bit longer and then you'll be able to go home. You'll have to fill out some paperwork first." With a grin and a swish of the curtain, he was gone. Worn out by all the unknowns, I asked the ultrasound tech to tell me the baby's sex: a boy.

Half an hour later, a new doctor, the attending who had taken over for my usual obstetrician, entered our little bunker. Over at the nurses' station, where the readings from my fetal cardiac machine were being monitored, the situation hadn't been evaluated with as much optimism as my physician had projected. This new doctor, who had a more brusque, direct manner, informed us that some abnormalities had been detected: the baby's heartbeat was a bit slow, and when it declined, it wasn't bouncing back as quickly it ought to. The technical terms zoomed over me, but instantly I could conjure a topographical image rendered by a heart monitor, the ones doctors had shown me when I was a teenager hospitalized for cardiac complications arising from my anorexia. The doctors' fingers would trace the line's decline and pause at the nadir: *Here*, they said then, *this is the junctional rhythm. It should begin pumping again sooner than it does.*

And now my baby's heart was mimicking that.

A maternal–fetal medicine specialist was quickly summoned. The doctors had formed a plan. They presented it to me tentatively, as if they were underlings offering up a presentation for their boss, fearful she might reject it: I would stay in the hospital, on a fetal cardiac monitor, for seven days, until I hit thirty-six weeks pregnant—that much closer to full-term. They would give me steroid shots to fast-track the baby's lung development, Pepcid to subdue the acid burning in my throat, ursodiol to bring the bile acids in my blood down, and prenatal vitamins, as if a last-minute dose of iron would quell whatever horrors were happening in my body. Then they would induce labor. If things went south, they could potentially induce labor earlier, even as early as that very day.

"Will the baby need to go to the neonatal intensive care unit?"

"Not necessarily," they said. "If he was born today, he would, because he would be under thirty-five weeks. But once you make it to thirty-five weeks, it would depend on need."

"How big is the baby now?" My older son, born at term, had been small, weighing in at five pounds eleven ounces, and in his early days we fretted often about his being tiny. I had originally hoped this baby would make it to at least six pounds.

"Four pounds, ten ounces," they said. My face sank, I'm sure. In response, they offered tentative optimism: "But if he's on track to gain an ounce a day, he could be five pounds by the time you deliver?" *If*, I thought: if he's on track, if we make it to next week, if we make it at all.

I reject this plan, I wanted to say. *Back to the drawing board.*

There was only one private room on the floor, so the team moved me to a bed in the recovery area; the curtain hung just a few inches from the perimeter of the bed, which made me claustrophobic, even though it didn't matter at all that there was no room to move because there was nowhere to go. Behind the other four or five curtains in the room, women who had just had c-sections were recuperating immediately following surgery. Oftentimes they had their babies with them, and I could hear the little ones yelping, followed by a parental coo or a nurse's *aww*. After I got settled in my bed, my husband went in to his office, so I was left alone with the most recent *New Yorker* and a promise of his quick return. I watched an article's words swirl on the page and then let it rest at my side. My gaze sometimes flickered to the fetal cardiac monitor. Two wide, sky-blue elastic bands, which were supposed to rest on my stomach, fed into the machine standing like a sentinel next to my bed. The machine had a screen on top, displaying a pair of numbers that rose and fell in some incomprehensible dance. It seemed a pretty crude instrument to be doing such delicate work. Sometimes a slight readjustment of my legs would cause the monitor to begin picking up my heartbeat instead of the baby's, subtly but unmistakably a louder and more forceful drumbeat. Heaven forbid I roll from one side to another, lest a frantic flurry of beeps ensue and cause my own heart rate to soar. Rarely did the nurses or physician's assistants seem to react to this with much concern; after a few minutes, someone would enter the room, shrug, readjust the machine, and then zip the curtain closed again. For the first few hours, I intently watched the numbers on the monitor, trying to decipher some code hidden within, until eventually I told myself that for the sake of my sanity, I had to do *literally* anything else.

Periodically someone would come in to give me a shot or to change my IV bag or hand me a little pleated white cup of pills. I abandoned all thought of reading and instead downloaded all nine seasons of *Everybody Loves Raymond*, a much-loved guilty pleasure, onto my computer. I let one episode slide seamlessly into another, sometimes drifting off into restless sleep, only occasionally taking out my headphones to hear an update from a doctor or answer a text. Once, I closed my computer for a bit to give my eyes a break from the blue light, only to overhear a conversation between a nurse and a new mother elsewhere in the room.

"Yeah, I mean, the emergency c-section was scary," the mom said. "And he's a little guy, so . . ."

"He's five pounds, eleven ounces!" the nurse said in response. "We have some term babies who are that big!"

I thought of my new child, as yet unnamed, whose existence felt not at all a sure bet at that moment, who would be lucky to weigh a full pound less. I silently cursed this woman, whose face I hadn't even seen.

/

"If everything continues this way, I think they'll let you go home today!" My cheerful nurse, Kristin, who had come on shift early in the morning of my second day at the hospital, seemed to think this news would enliven me, but I was shocked.

"Oh," I said. "I mean, that's great, but . . . I think I'll be scared . . . like, what if something goes wrong when I'm at home?"

"Don't worry," she said. "They're *very* careful. If they send you home, it means they're really confident. And you'll come back in frequently to get checked."

I envisioned myself sitting on the couch alone while my older son was at school, breathing heavily, my hands resting on my stomach as I waited for the faintest movement. Hours would pass that way. How could I ever do anything knowing that my activity might obscure some crucial sign from within? *Do you even* want *to go home?* I wondered, oddly accusatorily of myself. Of course, I did. But of course, I didn't. What I wanted wasn't so much for the situation to be made better but for it not to exist at all. I wanted to be having brunch with friends, whining about how the baby was keeping me up all night thrashing around, and *Oh my!* the doctors projected he'd be approaching eight pounds! And then I'd rub my burgeoning stomach and roll my eyes at how weird and exasperating and hilarious this whole pregnancy thing was.

I liked Kristin. She had caught me at the right moment: my husband had once again left for work, and I was lonely and longing for an ally. Kristin was sweet and went out of her way to help me, bringing me coffee when the hopelessly inept cafeteria lady forgot my order, sharing anecdotes about her own pregnancy, now twenty-five weeks along. I cringed a little when she complimented me on how small my bump was—surely, she must known I would have taken an extra fifty pounds over my current situation—but I decided to overlook that.

At other times, I would almost pick one of the nurses or physician's assistants at random and direct my frustration and anger at them, even though I knew it was unfair. In a moment, I would morph from the docile, obedient patient I'd always strived to be into her evil twin, the recalcitrant hospitalized anorexic—she only ever took the lead on rare occasions, even during the most defiant stage in my life—who bargained over a quarter slice of toast and lashed out when she wasn't allowed a paltry bit of agency. In the dead of the previous night, I had begged a physician's assistant to let me take off the monitor for two minutes, just so I could use the bathroom unfettered, but she had told me the whole point of being in the hospital was so I could be monitored, which I countered by telling her the monitor went off for up to a few minutes all the time and no one raced to turn it back on then, so they couldn't be *that* obsessed with monitoring me, to which she just repeated her first point, until I told her that was a *fucking ridiculous* argument, until finally she relented. When I came out of the bathroom, a baby wailed from down the hall, and I fell into bed sobbing because surely I would never meet my child, and she reminded me in a pissed-off tone that hospitals have *policies* and it's not to make the patients uncomfortable, it's for keeping us *safe* and—

"I'm not crying about that," I said, welling up again. "I'm crying about *the babies*." And that ended the conversation for good.

Still, as much as I liked Kristin, her good prognosis perplexed me. No other person at the hospital thus far had suggested that my going home was even a remote possibility. Not that everyone had prophesied doom, either. No, the reality was far more confusing than that: the assessments I had heard from the other nurses, doctors, maternal-fetal medicine specialists, and physician's assistants varied widely. One nurse would come tend to the machine after it had a beeping fit and tell me it was a technical error, only to be followed by a nurse who told me the baby's heart rate had, in fact, dipped in a worrying way. The baby's heart rate would be 100, and one nurse would raise her eyebrows to suggest that was too low, and then another would see it and brush it off as within normal range.

And on it went: one doctor would say things were staying stable, while another would suggest things seemed more tenuous. Sometimes a provider would use highly sophisticated medical language for a phenomenon occurring inside my or my baby's body—*variable decels, category 2 tracing, acontractile*—and then would be surprised when I said I'd never encountered that term before. Oftentimes, I would have to inform a physician of what a previous one had told me, and they'd check my file and concede that *Oh yes, that is, in fact, correct, my mistake.* Then I would get annoyed—shouldn't they be reading my chart carefully before talking to me, letting alone overseeing my care? Are these people just *making it up as they go along?*—before telling myself to consider how it must be impossible to keep everyone's stats straight especially when you work long hours and you have families of your own at home and you have needy patients who expect you to be thinking only of them every waking moment of your life. Other times I felt like my baby and I were the ones in a state of emergency, and all the other women on this floor were just having normal births and so wasn't I the one who deserved some clear answers—especially after all that time I spent trying to be an easy, low-maintenance patient? Of course I knew it wasn't their fault; I knew this wasn't *anyone's* fault. But I had so much directionless anger and sadness and confusion, and it had to go somewhere. Plus, my momentary eruptions made me feel, at times, that I was simply becoming a better advocate for myself in medical scenarios, a skill that I'd never quite mastered. Soon after my outbursts fizzled, I'd realize how futile they were, and how powerless many of the staff who tended to me actually were, and feel guilty.

On that second day, an attending physician I recognized from my obstetrician's practice came in and outlined the basics of what was happening for my husband and me, with no additional commentary.

"So, you're here for a week so the baby's heart can be monitored because the pulse is showing some irregularities."

"That's right."

"And you have a toddler at home."

"Yes."

"And we're giving you steroids for the lungs, and ursodiol for the cholestasis."

"Yes."

"And we'll wait and see where you are at thirty-six weeks."

"Yes."

"That's really hard. I'm sorry."

My husband gave him a death stare. "What do you mean by that?"

"Nothing," he said, shrugging. "That's really difficult. There's nothing else I can do other than watch you here. I'm just empathizing."

My initial rage evaporated when I realized he was doing what no one else in the hospital so far had done: acknowledging his limitations, and simply feeling sad for me.

Bless her heart, Kristin lobbied the other nurses to get me out of the recovery area, so in the early evening I moved down the hall to a sizable room with a wall-mounted TV, a private bathroom, and a little cot off to the side where my husband could sleep. After two days behind a curtain, I felt like I had been given the keys to a palace, blissfully distant from the assaulting cries of the babies and the sounds of the nurses joking with one another and the beeps from other people's machines, which I mistook for my own. That day was New York's only major winter storm that season, and outside my giant windows I could see the flurries swirl in the night sky. A friend who worked nearby visited: she shook the snow from her hair and presented me with books and magazines, gave me a quick hug and dashed off to her own children. The lights in the surrounding buildings turned off when the office workers went home, and for a moment, the whole set-up seemed peaceful, almost cozy. After a day or two, when I became more confident we'd make it to thirty-six weeks, I wondered if I could start to appreciate this time as a period of relaxation—a highly sterilized and monitored babymoon of sorts—before the hairy early newborn days.

I woke up at 4:30 that morning. A physician's assistant I didn't recognize was holding my shoulder.

"I'm sorry to wake you," she whispered. "Everything is fine, but I have to tell you that the baby's heart just experienced another decel—one of those big drops. I don't want you to panic, but I do think the powers-that-be should have a discussion this morning about what to do, because I have to be honest, I don't think you're going to make it another five days."

I started to cry.

"I know this is upsetting, but I didn't want you to be surprised later."

"What now?"

"Just try to go back to sleep. I'll be watching from the nurse's station. Your doctor is on today, so I'll call him and tell him what I think and have him come see you when he arrives."

Of course, I was already awake when the doctor walked in

and began shedding his civilian clothes. Untying his knotted scarf, he opened by telling me I needed to have my baby today.

"And I think you need to have a c-section. This baby is already stressed out, and if I put him through labor, he's going to end up in an emergency situation, and this is bad enough already as it is."

This was not good news: the last bit of hope I had for the situation was to avoid a c-section. I had always heard that the recoveries were worse than vaginal births—how would I handle a newborn and an active toddler post-surgery?

My husband's lawyerly urge to get all the facts kicked in. "Do we know if there is some holistic cause here? For example, is the cholestasis affecting the heartbeat …?"

"It wouldn't normally. Also, you know, fetal heart rate is not a great indicator of outcomes. The truth is that if you put a cardiac monitor on a person with no heart problems and you watched it all day, you'd probably see some wacky stuff. And cholesta-sis—even the correlation between cholestasis and stillbirth has been questioned in recent years. I had a patient recently who had cholestasis and I suggested she be induced and she said, 'No thanks, I'll take my chances,' and she ended up fine."

For a moment, I envisioned this woman: a brave birth war-rior woman, no doubt, an ideologue who refused to kowtow to medicine, whose reward for leading with principle was a magi-cal, empowering water birth in a bathtub surrounded by luxury candles, soft jazz playing in the background. Could this be the narrative: that I was led to this moment—to a manufactured, or at least overstated, crisis—by an absentminded cadre of doctors and nurses and assistants who couldn't even keep my diagnosis straight between them? But then I remembered the feeling of terror, my race up the stairs.

My doctor turned to address me directly. "You can refuse," he said.

I shook my head no. "We're not going to do that," my hus-band responded.

"Okay, but I have to give you the option. You can leave now, it's your right. But if you do, I won't be able to treat you any-more, because in my opinion it would be malpractice."

My husband's quest for a definitive source of the trouble—I'd long since given up on this—hadn't been sated. "But what could cause the reduction in movement?"

He shrugged again. "I am not sure. I was really scared when you guys came in, because there's no reason a fetus at this stage in a pregnancy would be moving less. I thought it was very likely the baby had died. But sometimes the cord wraps around the neck or the leg, or it gets clamped down in the armpit, and then the flow of oxygen is restricted and the heart rate drops. Or sometimes babies experience neurological issues, like a sei-zure in the womb"—the idea was so horrible, I immediately obliterated it, like an open palm slamming on an insect—"so that's why I'm hoping when we get in there, I'm going to see something with the cord."

My husband nodded, encouraged. I said nothing.

"Ultimately, I gotta tell you, obstetrics is not a great branch of medicine. We often have to weigh pros and cons of what we're seeing and make a guess. It's an educated guess, but it's still just a guess. This might be a really conservative move. In five months, you might be really angry with me for putting you through this. You might decide that it was totally unnecessary. But you know what? I don't care. All I care about is that you have your healthy baby in your arms."

Nobody said anything for a minute.

"I don't know why this happened," the doctor said. "I don't know how the cholestasis and the cardiac abnormalities relate to one another, or to the movement, or even if they relate."

He raised his palms upward toward the ceiling, in a gesture half-reverent, half-impotent. "All I can think is that the move-ments stopping was a sign from above, for you to get help."

/

My son was born on a chill November morning. He weighed four pounds and eleven ounces. In my drugged haze, I thought I heard my doctor mentioning something about the cord being under the baby's arm, but I couldn't be sure. My son's fragility and silence frightened me—I don't think he cried once during his first few days on earth—but he was, for all intents and purposes, healthy. Because he had spent thirty-five weeks and one day in the womb, he didn't have to go to the NICU automatically, but a few days after birth, he spent eighteen hours there due to a low body temperature. He was discharged from the hospital the same day I was. When we were getting ready to leave, I saw a blurry-eyed woman standing guard over one of the plastic NICU "habitats," as the nurses called them. It was the mother I had resented for having a bigger baby than I was projected to, just days earlier. Her son—Asher, Hebrew for *happy* or *blessed*—had been in the NICU that whole time, and had no forthcoming discharge date. For weeks after we left, I plotted ways to send her an anonymous gift as an apology—a teddy bear for the baby, maybe, or a platter with bagels and all the fixings—before realizing she'd have no idea who I was, or what I felt guilty for.

The next few weeks and months were a torturous blur of pumping-freezing-sterilizing-feeding-expressing-sleeping-sweating-pumping-freezing. Because my son was so tiny, the lactation consultant recommended pumping my breastmilk and then feeding the baby through a bottle, so he wouldn't have to work as hard and lose precious calories when he ate. I brought the baby to the pediatrician to be weighed twice a week, and it took all of my willpower not to pound on the office door demanding a weigh-in on the other days, too. Many days, it felt like all of my attention was focused on the ounces gained or lost, my mood determined solely by the numbers on the scale, as it had been, in a very different way, so many years ago. And my son slowly grew.

No root cause for my son's issues in utero have ever been

found. At my two-week follow-up with my obstetrician, he said my placenta had been deemed healthy by the pathology department at the hospital. This time, he seemed much more certain that my cholestasis was the cause of it all—"your bile acids were through the *roof*!" I wanted to ask him if he had remembered telling us that was unlikely, but I didn't, and to this day, I'm not exactly sure why, other than some part of me was still invested in being a complacent patient. He didn't mention the cord at all, and I didn't ask. Maybe it had been wrapped, and he forgot to mention it; maybe I had latched on to this possibly imaginary utterance as a simple, attractive explanation. I never even bothered to ask if the low PAPP-A could be linked to the birth, because I already knew the answer: *we just don't know.*

I have always felt like my doctor gave his rather poetic diagnosis—a literal divine intervention, which would have made an excellent note in my hospital charts—because he knew we were religious, and he figured it would comfort us. And yet I often wondered if he could have known that, despite being a person who cleaves to her faith, I often look around the world and don't see the unfolding of a plan devised by a wise, invisible force. Sometimes I think I do spot celestial workings, only to dismiss it later as randomness. When bad things happen to me, I'm almost never comforted by the concept that it's all part of intelligent machinations beyond our understanding: I pity myself, I wonder why it had to be like this, I obsess over whether I could have changed it. I cry out to my Creator all the time, I beg Him to intervene for me in matters big and small—maybe this is what makes me religious, that I cry to Him at all—but mostly, I feel alone.

And yet with an uncanny frequency, when I think about the birth and find myself tipping toward melancholy or weaving some conspiratorial tale about medical inadequacy, that randomness resurfaces in undeniably meaningful ways. I come across a stillbirth story—in a personal essay, maybe, or in a news article about pregnancy, or some anecdote buried in a celebrity profile—and I am shaken into gratitude by a glimpse of what could have been. When the doctor pronounces the baby dead in each story, I sob every time. And then I look down at the cheery, chubby infant at my feet and wonder what would have happened if I had waited to get help, if I had questioned my instinct and pushed it off as an overreaction for longer than I did. How long could he have lived—an hour, a day, a week? And then, having pushed myself as far toward the edge of that particular cliff as I'm willing to go, I'll scoop him up, nibble his soft neck, and crane back to watch him as he cackles with glee.

My son is more than a year old now. After months of vacillating between wildly divergent narratives, I've mostly accepted that the reality probably contains some of both: that it was a true emergency and I did the right thing, and that had I chosen a different kind of birthing path, some aspects of the experience could have been better. I do still occasionally search for the root cause of his problems in utero—scanning his face for the lingering signs of a neurological trauma, seeing every sniffle, every rash as the key to unlocking that original, inscrutable enigma. And I still wonder if things could have been different if I had held out a bit longer: If I had a term baby, a five-pound baby, would I feel more confident—in him, in myself? The trauma of all the unanswered questions is usually drowned out by the (mostly) joyful chaos of life with two toddlers. But sometimes, when I am motionless, I feel a little twitch in my stomach—a minor digestive reaction, or a muscular spasm, some kind of phantom quickening. A slight panic detonates within, until I remember that I am not pregnant anymore; there is no baby inside who needs saving. And yet even now, in those moments, I feel compelled to say *something*, to commemorate the time when the fear was real and the child was in peril, even if we still don't know how. At once helplessly and courageously, I call out to that still, small voice: *I am here. I am listening.*

My Cross-Continental Miracle

BY PRAMILA JAYAPAL

Having a child prematurely is the ultimate reminder of the uncertainty of life. All parents of young children come to learn this in some form—but perhaps parents with challenging early experiences with parenthood understand very quickly that you simply cannot control everything, regardless of how much planning you do. You just have to take life as it comes.

Nothing about the birth of my first and only child went according to my carefully plotted plan: Janak Jayapal Preston was born on February 27, 1997, in Mumbai, India, at only twenty-seven and a half weeks and weighed just one pound, fourteen ounces.

In 1982, at the age of sixteen, I had moved to the United States by myself for college. I would spend the next eighteen years on an alphabet soup of student and work visas in order to stay in the country. I began working in the private sector, but in 1991, I moved to Seattle to work for an international nonprofit organization focused on global public health and development. That work—traveling in and around many parts of the world, including India—made me long to return to India to explore my own identity, to ground myself in who I was and where I came from, and to figure out if I was Indian, American, or something else. And so I applied for and was granted a fellowship from the Institute of Current World Affairs to return to India—my birth country—to live, write, and research in its small towns and villages.

Being back in India changed me in so many ways. India is a place of contradictions: I saw overwhelming poverty and unbearable sadness but also love, generosity, resilience, community, and fellowship. I had the opportunity to tap back into a lineage of powerful Indian women leaders: from my mother, grandmother, and great-aunt to the forest-saving village women and young village girls I met. I reconnected to a power that would be central to my identity long into the future. Being in India brought me back to who I was as an Indian and as an American.

Alan, my husband at the time, and I knew we wanted to have a baby, and we thought we had the perfect plan: I would get pregnant just before I finished my fellowship in India, then return to the United States for the third trimester and birth—which would also put us back in the country in just enough time to keep my green card, or Lawful Permanent Resident immigration status, current.

Being pregnant in India was its own journey. Pregnancy was treated extremely differently depending on your class. In the United States, most of my friends who were pregnant carried on their lives as usual—going to their jobs and keeping up regular exercise until just before their deliveries. In India, concerned friends told me I should not ride in a rickshaw or carry even a single bag of groceries home. It was expected that upper-middle-class or middle-class women would go on complete bed rest during their pregnancy, moving in with their mothers, doing very little work, and receiving daily oil massages. Meanwhile, poorer women's work continued as usual with little relief, leave, or even a change of duties to accommodate for the pregnancy. Similar to what we see in America, low-wage workers are essential but do not get the most basic of rights: sufficient wages, paid leave, access to health care, or basic public health protections in dire situations. This hypocrisy only comes to light even more during crises, like the COVID-19 pandemic.

I did not want to be treated differently or make a fuss over my pregnancy. I wanted to carry on with life as usual, which included living in villages with little electricity or few other comforts and continuing to take those bumpy rickshaw rides on potholed streets.

I did, however, want to find a really good gynecologist—a task that was far harder than I expected. Many of them operated according to the model of "doctor knows best," with too little information for the patient. That wouldn't do for me. I went through a long search before finding Dr. Prakash, who would turn out to be a literal lifesaver.

Everything seemed to be proceeding according to plan until two weeks before we were scheduled to return to the United States. I was nearly twenty-six weeks pregnant when I suddenly developed a leak in my amniotic sac. I called Dr. Prakash, who prescribed immediate bed rest to see if the leaking would stop. He impressed upon me the fact that saving a baby this premature is difficult anywhere in the world. In Varanasi, where we were living at the time, there was no advanced medical technology or infrastructure, making it virtually impossible.

I decamped to bed as Alan finished packing up boxes, hopefully to return to the United States in just weeks. At the time, we were living in a small apartment up a long flight of stairs. We had no car or phone, although our landlady downstairs was generous if we needed to use her phone. The nearest medical clinic was across town on bumpy, crowded roads, so Dr. Prakash was hesitant to send me unless it was absolutely necessary. After a week of trying to buy time, however, the leaking had not stopped and Dr. Prakash sent me across town to get an ultrasound. The ultrasound showed that only half of the amniotic fluid that cushions and nourishes a baby in utero remained, and the weight of the baby was just one-point-one kilograms, or a little less than two and half pounds—a dangerously low weight.

If the baby were to have even a small chance of survival, I needed to have a c-section immediately—which meant we had to leave Varanasi and fly to one of the only two neonatal intensive care units in the country that would be somewhat equipped to handle such a low-birthweight baby—if the baby even survived that long.

The next days proceeded in a blur. Quickly, we had to find someone willing to deliver the baby—many doctors refused because of the tremendous precariousness of such a premature birth—and fly to either Mumbai or Delhi. We finally secured a gynecologist in Mumbai connected to the NICU that had just been established in a very good hospital. Of course, the car we ordered did not arrive because of massive student protests that had broken out and blocked the roads. I was quickly bundled into a friend's van and driven through the middle of riots in the streets, only to arrive at the airport just as the plane pulled away from the gate.

I spent a painful night of more leaking in a hotel near the airport, until the next flight the following morning. Just after takeoff, I noticed that I had started bleeding. Terrified, Alan arranged to have an ambulance meet us at the airport and transport us to the hospital to perform the c-section immediately. I went under around 10:45 p.m. When I woke up, my husband told me the news: Our baby was alive. Janak was alive.

I was weak from surgery, but I had to see my miracle child. I will never forget that first look: Janak in an infant warmer, weighted down with IVs, so tiny that they fit neatly in the palm of my hand, just skin and bones and a head larger than their body. In spite of all of it, our baby was alive and beautiful.

Over the next two and a half months, we visited the NICU every day. We would hold fiercely to Janak's tiny fingers as nurses pricked our baby with needles, clamped devices on their arms and legs to measure blood pressure and oxygen levels, and stuck ECG leads on their chest. The NICU was brand new, and Janak was the lowest-birthweight baby to be born there. That posed challenges as well. The simple but effective practice of "kangaroo care"—putting a baby directly onto the parents' chests for skin-to-skin contact several hours every day as a way to give the baby a sense of security and to increase bonding between parent and child—was not known and was frowned upon by the nurses. It took me some time to convince everyone that this was an important practice that would benefit the baby's health. Getting the necessary medications was also challenging because they were expensive and not stocked by the hospital. Alan and I would take rickshaws at all hours of day and night to find the necessary medications from various twenty-four-hour pharmacies.

My inability to breastfeed plagued me. Janak was born so early that they had no muscles formed in their mouth to be able to suckle, and few digestive organs to process any amount of milk. The dominant culture around us all, around the world, ties "good mothering" to breastfeeding. The nurses in the brand-new NICU didn't understand fully the mechanics of breastfeeding and preemies, and they constantly made remarks that left me feeling ashamed I could not breastfeed. These stereotypes of "good mothering" are ones that I have heard many parents of premature babies over the years raise. The internal and external oppressions from societal expectations can be severe when a birth does not go according to plan.

Janak needed a total of seven blood transfusions. At one point, the hospital had no blood left to give to our baby, so our pediatrician gave his own blood. I cannot overstate how lucky we were—to have given birth in the best hospital in Mumbai and, especially, to have Dr. Mahesh Baleskar as our pediatrician. Dr. Baleskar took it upon himself to be more than a doctor to us. He and his wife befriended and took care of me and Alan, making sure we took breaks from the round-the-clock vigilance Janak's care required, inviting us to attend a concert with him, making themselves available to us, for anything, day or night.

I carefully tracked every development, from the number of grams my baby weighed to the days I could breastfeed any amount of milk successfully. Progress was achingly slow.

It took a full month to know that Janak would actually live— and for that, we gave enormous thanks. But the medical needs were still tremendous and Janak was in critical condition; it simply was not clear just what kind of life our child would be able to have.

As Janak's situation developed additional complexities, we faced real challenges: the Indian hospital's technology, equipment, and even some of their knowledge about low-birthweight babies was still new and limited. In addition to the enormous medical concerns, there were logistical ones. In order to preserve my permanent resident status, I would have needed to return to the United States within weeks of giving birth. But returning would mean leaving Janak, who faced down death every single day for months. I refused to leave their side, knowing that they might die. If I had to lose my green card because of that, and my ability to return to the United States with my family, so be it.

Alan was outraged. He was a U.S. citizen and by that virtue so was our child, but I—as the mother—was going to be denied reentry to the country because our baby was too sick for me to leave? That meant even as we fought to keep Janak alive every single day, we also had to worry about how we could keep our family together. In the end, we were enormously fortunate. Through my fellowship, we were able to contact officials at the U.S. Embassy and plead our case directly. Back then, the United States was far more compassionate to special circumstances than the cruelty of its policies under the Trump administration, for instance.

In the end, I was able to get my green card reinstated so I could return to the United States, but all the years that had accumulated to make me eligible for my citizenship were wiped away and I would need to wait another three years to qualify again for U.S. citizenship. The fear that I would be separated from my child and family because of my immigration status, the dependence on the benevolence of U.S. immigration officials, and all of the deep stresses that come with having a premature baby in a place with few resources for preemie births created visceral emotions that stayed with me for decades. These feelings often resurfaced when I addressed the plight of immigrant moms who had been separated from their children, or families that could not be together.

By June 1997, more than three months after Janak's delivery, we finally did return to the United States. However, my tiny baby's trauma—and mine—was far from over. Janak developed hydrocephalus, or water in the brain, and needed to be seen by a neurosurgeon within two days of returning to Seattle. Fortunately, they did not ultimately need surgery. There were also yearly bouts of pneumonia and constant fears of developmental delays. One day, Janak had a terrifying seizure when we were at home alone.

Navigating the medical system in this intense way, across two continents, requires constant self-advocacy. For all the toll it took on me, I was able to do it because of many privileges. In India, I had money for the best doctors and the necessary medications. But I saw how hard it was to communicate in a country where I did not speak the language as well as I needed to in all situations. What if I hadn't been able to speak the language at all? How would I have managed? How do all of the immigrants in this country manage in such a situation? What if I hadn't known *how* to advocate for the best care, or ask the right questions of my doctors?

I was and am today all too aware that Janak's survival depended on our income and insurance. My fellowship covered all medical expenses while in India, and the Institute arranged for excellent health insurance once I returned to the United States. I had choices that so many families don't get when a premature birth occurs. More babies are born prematurely in the United States than in other industrialized countries, and studies have shown that lack of access to affordable health care is a huge risk factor—nearly 20 percent of uninsured women deliver preterm.* In fact, many of the troubling trends in preterm birth rates in the United States track with so many other devastating health disparities in our broken system. We also have some of

---

* Christopher Ingraham, "Lack of Access to Health Insurance Keeps U.S. Premature Birth Rate Near Somalia's," *The Washington Post*, November 13, 2014.

the highest maternal mortality and infant mortality rates, and they are three times worse for women of color. African American women, in particular, have the highest preterm birth rate of any ethnicity, at 13.6 percent.*

I firmly believe that health care is a human right. Everyone, no matter who they are, should be able to get the care they need—including emergency care, maternity care, and the life-saving and expensive procedures Janak needed—without worrying about affording it or having to give up their housing to pay medical expenses. The work I had been doing for years before Janak's birth to advance reproductive and maternal health for women in countries across Asia, Latin America, and Africa became very real and personal for me. My experience added one more arrow in my quiver of reasons for why health care is absolutely essential for any life of dignity, and for everything else in our lives to work.

That's partly why I am the proud lead author of the bill in the House of Representatives. It's why I worked with a diverse coalition of health care providers, labor groups, and advocates to get the largest, most comprehensive Medicare for All bill its first prime-time hearings in 2019—the first ever in the history of Congress. My Medicare for All bill actually lowers and contains overall health care costs by cutting administrative waste. Whenever you may be reading this, I hope that we have moved to a system that guarantees barriers to quality health care are a thing of the past—that guarantees health care for all.

The average cost of giving birth in the United States is $4,000—more than many Americans have in their savings accounts at any given time.** For a preterm birth, the cost is $65,000, and many NICU bills soar far higher. Medicare for All

---

* March of Dimes 2019 Report Card. Accessed at https://www. marchofdimes.org/mission/reportcard.aspx

** March of Dimes 2016 Report Card. Accessed at https://www. marchofdimes.org/materials/premature-birth-report-card- united-states.pdf

would make sure no one pays debilitating premiums, deductibles, or copays. Procedures to save a parent's or an infant's life should be accessible, affordable, and include explicit nondiscrimination protections; employers and providers should not be able to opt out of providing a particular procedure. Universal, guaranteed health care for everyone; no co-pays, premiums, or deductibles, no surprise bills, no profit-making motives that drive costs up. Just health care, guaranteed. Everybody in, nobody out. No parent, dealing with the challenges of birth and premature birth in particular, should ever have to worry about whether they can get the care they need, whether their baby will get the care necessary for a strong recovery, or have to deal with the anxiety of costs and everything else. There is so much to worry about with prematurity; no one should have to worry about cost on top of it.

Even with luck, resources, and self-advocacy, of course, Janak and I were not spared the mental and emotional toll of our birth experience. It was a profoundly lonely experience. I had been used to bustling communities in India where friends dropped by for tea. American culture felt so isolated in comparison. Back in Seattle, it felt as though the friends I made before I left for India had moved on with their lives and did not have much energy for a friend with a brand-new, very vulnerable baby. I did not realize until talking with a therapist years later that I suffered from postpartum depression and post-traumatic stress disorder in the months and years following the birth.

The depression made me feel like a failure on many levels. Depression so often arises beneath the weight of cultural expectations. There is a built-in expectation, an idealized vision of parenthood that is joyful and perfect, where the parent is full of constant love and affection for their child, breastfeeds with ease, and wants to be with their child at every moment. It felt as though there was no room to talk about the real feelings that happen in pregnancy and early parenthood, some of which are hormonal and others that come with the big shift in our life and in our identity. There was no room to discuss the different realities for difficult, extremely premature births. This kind of pressure can also be devastating and difficult for families to weather together. A few years after Janak's birth, I went through a painful divorce which, while not directly attributable to the trauma of the birth, compounded my feelings of inadequacy.

All of this also affected my relationship with Janak. It took a lot of time to process fully and come to terms with the fact that I did not have a perfect birth—and that was neither my failure nor Janak's. Our relationship was rocky at times, but through deep, honest conversation and listening to each other, we have forged a beautiful relationship of closeness and understanding. At twenty-three, Janak is even more of a miracle child than at birth. They have become a friend and even a teacher in matters of gender, sexuality, race, and the changing norms of any society in transition. Several years ago, Janak came out as nonbinary. I saw in them the joy of openly being who they are; and I easily embraced their full identity, although I had to train myself to change habits and use new pronouns and other language with intentionality.

Today, Janak is my great pride. I have watched them flourish and thrive as a thinker, musician, and hobby chef. They have continued to discover newly released creativity, resilience, and freedom in not having to hide parts of themselves. Even as they create new music, they are deeply engaged in social change work and movements. They are organized, practical, and resilient in a way that children can only be when they have had to weather storms at early ages.

My birth experience was deeply challenging. Learning to trust myself as a mother and accept the unexpected challenges of a premature birth was perhaps a strange gift, though I couldn't see it as such for many years. But what is strength except that which emerges in times of crisis? The things I fight for today— the right to make choices about one's own body, universal health care and child care, immigration reform that keeps families together—in some way all had roots in this birth.

And yes, I do completely believe in miracles, because by all medical standards, Janak should not be alive today. And yet, here they are thriving and joining me in pushing for a more just, inclusive future.

What We Made

BY SARAH DIGREGORIO

On the third day after my daughter was born—what they called "day three of life" in that strange and particular neonatal intensive care unit jargon—a nurse showed me the breast-milk pumping room. I shuffled after her with difficulty, wearing a cotton hospital gown and wheeling a butter-yellow industrial-grade pump behind me. Next to the closet, where everyone kept their coats, there was a door with a keypad. The password was, I believe, 1234. Inside the small, windowless room were two chairs facing each other, and a sink with a soap dispenser and paper towels in one corner. On the wall, a bulletin board explained preemie care basics, like how to use cupped hands to cradle your baby's body, firm and still like the muscular walls of a uterus. The pumping room was the size of a very large walk-in closet or a very small kitchen. If you sat in one chair, you could lean forward and touch the other.

Parents needed a designated place to pump milk because our NICU was an open ward: several rooms lined with incubators, each just a few feet away from the next, and there was no other private space—not that this space could exactly be called private. I hated it the minute I saw it.

The nurse made sure I understood what to do and then said she'd give me some time. It was obvious that all of the doctors and nurses really wanted me to pump, though they pushed it gently and kindly. They said it was better, much better, for premature babies to get breast milk than formula, that my milk was the most important thing I could give her. I gathered that my daughter, Mira, would be less likely to die if I could manage to use this machine to wring some milk out of myself. (In the years since, donor breast milk has become more available for the most vulnerable premature babies, if their parents can't or don't want to pump.) I felt I had failed at every other bodily task, having produced a baby smaller than a rotisserie chicken, whose future was unknowable. So I was an easy sell, desperate to give Mira something of myself.

I felt utterly alone in this, but in fact, my feelings were not at all unique. One study[*] on what pumping breast milk means to mothers in a NICU found that *most* women had close-to-the-bone, strongly conflicting emotions about pumping: that it held both power and powerlessness, the feeling of being a mother and the feeling of not being a mother. When you have a baby who cannot eat by mouth, of course, pumping is a choice you can make, but it is also not really a *choice*. Feeding by tube, whether with milk or formula, is not how anyone envisions nourishing their baby. In that study, Linda Sweet, an Australian professor of midwifery, wrote of mothers' feelings on the matter: "The breast milk offered a means of connection to the baby, but only after disconnection of the mother and baby and the mother and her milk. They desired physical closeness and something special from their breastfeeding experience, but they were only able to have technical provision with mechanical equipment." This rings true. I was the only mother Mira had, so only I could give her breast milk. But I needed a battalion of professionals and technology to give it to her on my behalf: connection and disconnection. A machine-made closeness; a miracle and a rending.

The pump itself, the one I was renting from the hospital, looked a little like an oblong kettlebell, hefty and sleek. The model was called a Symphony, a name so dissonant with the

---

[*] L. Sweet, "Expressed Breast Milk as 'Connection' and Its Influence on the Construction of 'Motherhood' for Mothers of Preterm Infants: A Qualitative Study," *International Breastfeeding Journal* 3, 30 (2008), https://doi.org/10.1186/1746-4358-3-30.

reality that you almost had to admire it. Sitting in the pumping room, I fumbled with the pump pieces. Push the plastic bit with the flappy rubber membrane into the bottom of the valve and then screw the valve onto a bottle. Push the flange—the conical part that goes over your breast—into the other end of the valve. Press one end of the thin clear plastic tube into the back of the valve, and the other end into the top of the pump. Repeat. I hadn't gotten a pumping bra yet, so instead I pulled my hospital gown apart, and just held the flanges against my breasts, awkwardly, and started the pump. It spooled up with a rhythmic wheeze-groan-wheeze-groan. I started to cry.

The door swung open. It was another mom in regular street clothes, wheeling her own pump. Her glance slid over me in a practiced way and she gave me a small smile while also managing to give me privacy. She planted herself in the other chair and expertly hooked herself up, her hands swift and adept. "You need to get a pumping bra," she said. I nodded and blinked, lacking a free hand to wipe my eyes. She asked how old my baby was. How many weeks; how big. The relevant stats in this world.

Three days, I said. Twenty-eight weeks. 720 grams today. Intrauterine growth restriction.

She nodded, unsurprised. When I had told friends and relatives this information about Mira, there were terrible shocked silences. But this was normal to her. She had had IUGR too, she said. Her baby was born around the same size and gestation, and she said they were going home soon. "It'll happen," she said. "It'll happen before you know it."

No one had said anything remotely like this to me yet. From the professionals, it was all caution: "We'll see how she does"; "We don't want her to lose more weight"; "We're taking it day by day." This woman's confidence was incredible to me. At that moment, I didn't believe her. But her words landed and stuck. She was a future to imagine and to hope for. One without uncontrollable crying jags. One in which I would wear regular clothes again and know how to use the stupid pump. We would take our baby home and this would be over. I never forgot what she said, and the surety with which she said it.

The pumping room was small and crowded because everything in New York City is small and crowded, and there's an art to sharing space with many people. There was a certain etiquette to the pumping room that we learned by practice and observation, not unlike the subway. We all found ways to acknowledge each other politely without making full eye contact or imposing too much of ourselves on each other. If you could wait until someone was finished before you came in, you did. If someone was crying but didn't seem to want to talk, we didn't talk. If the other person gave a subtle cue that they might want to chat, it was polite to ask about their baby—those NICU stats becoming our own shorthand—but not to push for details. We all agreed to ignore the fact that our boobs were hanging out. It was not polite to comment on the quantity of milk pumped by someone else, although self-disparaging remarks about one's own low yield were common.

No one, of course, was happy to be there. We were parents hooked up to machines; our babies were hooked up to machines. All of those machines were replacements for what our bodies would have been doing, under different circumstances. The technology breathed for my baby, cradled my baby, and kept her warm. The machines sucked the milk out of my body and dripped it into hers. Sometimes I closed my eyes while pumping and imagined my body still connected to hers by a cord, a tube, anything.

In the pumping room, we were all trying to figure out how to live this way. To me, everything felt perilous. The closeness of other bodies and breath, the milk itself destined for Mira's fragile body, the chair and surfaces we all shared—who had touched them? Where had they been? What did they carry? The pumping room brought out the worst of my postpartum anxiety and OCD. I'd scrub the sink area with disinfectant over and over. I'd lay fresh paper towels out on the counter, let the water run and run until it got as hot as possible and then scrub the pump pieces with soap before gingerly placing them on the covered counter. But nothing was ever clean enough, safe enough. The paper towels were the dark brown kind that come out in an accordion fold, smell like dirt, and disintegrate the minute they get wet. The water didn't get that hot. I had put Mira here in this place, in danger, by having a body that couldn't do its job, and now I feared I would somehow poison her with my contaminated milk. It was not possible to be careful enough.

No one ever called me out on my obsessive behavior in that tiny room; no one ever reacted when I shot them a dirty look after they sneezed. We had all come apart in our own ways.

Weeks ticked by, and I would soon open the pumping room door to discover former versions of myself—weepy newbies in hospital gowns fumbling with the pump pieces—and realize that little by little, I was becoming more like the woman reporting confidently from the future. That was how the pumping room worked.

But these kinds of shared pumping rooms are vanishing as many NICUs transition to private patient rooms, one for each baby. Should we mourn the quiet passing of a space no one wants to be in?

When babies are cared for in individual rooms, parents benefit from having private space with their babies—they can have their own chairs, and sometimes even beds for sleeping over. They can shut the door or pull a curtain and pump next to their baby, by themselves. There are lots of advantages to this, advantages I can imagine personally—more protection and comfort, calm and control—and advantages that are documented in the scientific literature[*]: fewer complications, shorter stays, more family involvement and satisfaction.

---

[*] N. O'Callaghan, A. Dee, and R. K. Philip, "Evidence-based Design for Neonatal Units: A Systematic Review." *Maternal Health, Neonatology and Perinatology* 5, 6 (2019). https://doi.org/10.1186/s40748-019-0101-0

I would have loved to be able to close a door to pump, or just be alone with Mira. In this, also, I was not unusual. Researchers examining how NICU design affects parents' lactation experiences found that many parents strongly prefer private family rooms, in part because they would rather pump in a private room with their baby than in a shared pumping room.* It's easier, and they believe they produce more milk that way.

But private rooms are not a panacea—there's also some evidence** that language delays might be more common in preemies who were cared for in private rooms. And research also illuminates something that will be no surprise to anyone who has had to pump in a NICU: parents almost invariably struggled with pumping, no matter what kind of room their babies had. Pumping is full of obstacles: logistical, physical, and emotional. And, as always, those obstacles are compounded for those affected by racism, income inequality, and other kinds of marginalization.

Still, private rooms do ease some of the burdens of pumping. And family-centric, thoughtful NICU design can be helpful in many ways. Often, parents have access to support groups or lactation consultants, and all of the supplies they need to keep their pump pieces clean and organized. Some hospitals even offer lactating parents three meals a day in shared spaces, which is also a low-pressure opportunity to chat. This rethinking of the physical NICU organization—coupling more privacy with options for connection and support—is likely the best solution for reducing stress on parents and babies alike.

---

*   Dr. Donna A. Dowling and Mary Ann Blatz at Case Western Reserve University and Rainbow Babies & Children's Hospital, interview with the author, March 16, 2020.

** R. G. Pineda, J. Neil, D. Dierker, et al., "Alterations in Brain Structure and Neurodevelopmental Outcome in Preterm Infants Hospitalized in Different Neonatal Intensive Care Unit Environments." *The Journal of Pediatrics*, 164(1):52–60.e2 (2014). https://doi.org/10.1016/j.jpeds.2013.08.047

But I don't want to let the shared pumping room vanish without acknowledging its unexpected gifts, its ragged intimacy. I am surprised that I do, actually, mourn its passing. Without the pumping room, I would not have met that woman from the future, the first person to express confidence in Mira. Because of the pumping room, I didn't need anyone to tell me that pumping is really hard—that it wasn't just me—because I could see that it was different for everyone and easy for no one. I didn't need anyone to tell me that it was common to be weepy, irritable, confused, or afraid, because I saw that, too. There were no professionals there; it was just us, which meant that no one was managing or conveying information or calling us "Mom." It was an honest place.

If Mira had been in a private room, I could have gotten similar information at a support group in the hospital—and there are also online support groups, through groups like Hand to Hold. Those options are very important. But the truth is, I didn't *want* to go to a support group—I was afraid of what I might hear or feel. And it would have required me to make time and space that I felt I didn't have. The fact that the pumping room could not be avoided was why I hated it, but it's also why it was necessary: to orient, to contextualize.

The pumping room was not like a support group—we were not necessarily *trying* to support each other. We were not even really becoming friends. We were just doing what we had to do: pump every three hours so that a nurse could drip a few milliliters of our milk through our babies' feeding tubes. In this room, at least, no one was shocked by any of it. No one's mouth dropped open on learning your baby's weight. No one said, "I had no idea a baby that small could live." It was the everyday reality of our bodies, and the everyday conversations that we had to distract ourselves from those bodies. It was the small talk after the customary NICU stats had been exchanged. I chatted with one woman about her dog and about the logistics of applying for maternity leave all of a sudden and months too soon. I talked to another woman about her work, writing young adult fantasy. I talked to another about the restorative soups her mother-in-law made for her. To do this, we had to summon something of ourselves from the before-time, our identities outside this place. It was a reminder that I *could* still conjure myself, from the large to the small aspects of who I was and what I was experiencing: I'm an editor at a magazine; I liked this podcast; I enjoyed this book; I found this super-cheap parking lot close to the hospital.

When I think about the pumping room now, I know the difficulty and sorrow contained there. I wouldn't want to go back. But in hindsight, it's easier to see its beauty. Actually, it's easier to see *our* beauty. We were constructing our own motherhood in that bare little room. It wasn't the kind of motherhood we wanted, but it was the one we had. We were making it out of whole cloth. We were showing each other how. We were trying and failing. We were bleeding. We were saving what could be saved. We were showing each other a future.

Mama Knows Best?

BY MELODY SCHREIBER

In the beginning, "Mama" is aspirational. Anticipatory. You clutch the slender pregnancy test, you watch the tiny pulsating heart on the ultrasound, you spread your fingers over your growing belly and you think, *I'm going to be a mom.* It's thrilling in its distance; you have time, still, to become that person. To become someone else. Someone's *mother.*

They start calling you Mom in labor and delivery. The techs, nurses, doctors, and specialists all bustle in—*Hello Mom, Hi Mama, I'm here to draw blood, Here are your meds, I wanted to chat about what will happen when your little one arrives.* At first, confused, you look around for your own mother. Then you realize: No. It's you.

Perhaps no one feels ready when the water breaks, when the contractions start, when the adoption paperwork comes through. But you really thought you'd have more time. You had another trimester to check off; your baby registry, whenever you logged in, reminded you that delivery was a comfortable twelve weeks away.

Mama, we confirmed that it was amniotic fluid you felt. Mama, we're going to give you a shot to help the baby's lungs in case he arrives soon. Mama, you're doing great. Just keep that baby inside you. It's a way to be friendly without being specific; after a while, you stop correcting them with your own name and you just nod. You suspect they also call you Mama to get you used to the idea of becoming a parent, now, three months earlier than you expected. If only the rest of parenthood would come so effortlessly, simply by naming it.

And when the baby does arrive, tiny as a hollow-boned bird, you hold him to your chest and you wish you could do this next part for him. If only you could change places; he could go home with his father and you would gladly stay in the hospital for weeks, months, enduring the endless blood draws and procedures and the tubes threaded throughout your entire body, a second set of lungs, a second circulatory system, a second life to keep you tethered to this one.

But you're a mother now. Your first lesson is about separation. The doctor gently lifts the baby from your arms and sets him in his minuscule hospital bed to be wheeled off to intensive care.

/

This is the story of everything we didn't expect.

It had only been a few hours, but already my son's birth seemed so distant. He was now connected to everything but me, it seemed—tubes to breathe and to eat, heart monitors and pulse oximeters and arterial IVs taped to splints on his tiny limbs.

"He looks like he was in a car crash," Jack, my husband, murmured next to me.

Our baby was born twenty-nine weeks and six days into my pregnancy. At three pounds, seven-point-seven ounces, he was both bigger than we'd expected and smaller than seemed possible. His legs were little sticks, devoid of any baby fat. His fingers and toes were so narrow, they looked translucent; it seemed like they would snap in two at any touch. His skin was already covered in bruises from IV insertions and blood draws. His ears were as soft and slack as flower petals; they hadn't developed collagen yet. He had no eyelashes; his eyes, when they finally opened, were inky black.

He was absolutely beautiful.

I reached out a finger and stroked our baby's tiny belly, which was the size of the palm of my hand. Beyond that, though, I had no idea what to do. I'd been around countless babies before;

my parents had eleven children in all, and I had grown up with siblings and nieces and nephews all around me. Premature birth had always been with us, too, looming in the background. When I was four years old, my twin sisters were born at twenty-six weeks. They soon passed away from heart and lung complications, and the grief ricocheted throughout my family for decades. From the time I'd checked into the hospital two weeks earlier, my parents and siblings had feared for me and the baby.

At such a young gestational age, my son was too tiny to breastfeed; instead, my breast milk, fortified with extra calories, dripped into his stomach through a feeding tube. We couldn't even hold him for the first few weeks. First a ventilator and then a CPAP tube covered his mouth and nose to push oxygen into his lungs, making it difficult to move him; and dislodging his arterial IV could make him bleed out in a few horrific moments.

Around me, the nurses and doctors of the neonatal intensive care unit bustled and buzzed with practiced efficiency. They knew far more about what was happening with my own baby than I did—yet hadn't I grown him in my own body? Hadn't I talked to him late at night and promised that I would do anything I could to protect him? That had to count for something. Didn't it? But promises aren't medical expertise. His life was in their hands, not mine.

The next day, I left the hospital for the first time in what felt like years. After my water had broken spontaneously, I'd stayed on strict hospital bed rest for eighteen days, surrounded by monitors tracking my health and the baby's. The world felt different now: brighter and more demanding, yet harder to focus; louder, yet indistinct. Spring moved crisply through the air, blooming flowers and damp earth. My husband pulled our car out of the hospital parking lot and onto the freeway ramp to go home, and I felt a sudden sharp ache blossom in me. I wanted to claw at the car door and scream, "No, no, we have to go back! *We forgot the baby!*"

But we kept driving, farther and farther away.

At home, I was met with weeks of work that had gone unfinished while I was on bed rest. The nursery was a jumble of hastily stored items I'd acquired during pregnancy; we needed to assemble a crib, needed to unpack and organize boxes of clothes and toys and baby gear. I needed to figure out my new breast pump; I needed to figure out what our life was going to be like now.

But being at home meant counting down the minutes until I could return to the NICU. Home was just a place to sleep and pump; the rest of the time, I wanted to be at my baby's side. Yet there was nothing I could do for him there; I couldn't even hold him. Instead, I pressed my forehead against the plastic walls of his isolette and I whispered promises: *We're going to be okay. Everything will be fine.*

I had no idea if these were my first lies to him.

A few nights later, a friend came over to our house for dinner. Afterward, we sat around the table playing cards, just like we had on game nights before. It was like nothing had happened; like my baby had disappeared as soon as my belly deflated. Our lives were supposed to change with a baby. What did it mean that we could just go back to our lives as if he never existed? What kind of parents were we?

But, of course, we hadn't gone back to normal. We were in limbo. Purgatory. We had to prove ourselves before we could bring our baby home.

At every diaper change, every temperature check, we were becoming parents in front of a crowd of professionals. All of our early memories are set to the flashing lights and beeping soundtrack of a hospital intensive care unit, the sharp smell of antiseptic, the cries of other babies and the murmurs of other parents and nurses. The first time I breastfed my son—finally! joyously!—a little movable wall afforded me the only measure of privacy. Nurses and lactation consultants surrounded us, monitoring the baby, correcting my technique.

But breastfeeding, of course, was still far in the future. For now, I pumped militantly, manically. I set alarms to remind myself to pump every two or three hours; I kept meticulous records of dates and times and milliliters. At night, sometimes having a baby seemed theoretical, hypothetical. I wondered once, in a sleep-deprived haze, if other parents ever slept through their alarms, too, and then I remembered that their babies were there to wake them. I was tethered not to a baby but to an alarm and a pump, weak technological stand-ins for my son. Instead of watching my baby nurse, I gripped the double pumping cones and lost myself in thirty-minute increments of mindless television so I wouldn't think, in those raw, bare hours, of how much I missed him, the baby who had never been in this home. But still I pumped. This was the only thing I could really do for him.

A week after our son was born, the neonatologist detected a murmur in his heartbeat. The doctor ordered an echocardiogram, and the results showed a medium-sized hole in our tiny baby's heart. My husband and I were bereft, rocked into silence. The doctor assured us that most of these cases resolved themselves; but if not, in a year or so we could undergo a fairly noninvasive procedure to patch the hole. Until then, he said, the baby was asymptomatic. There was no use worrying about this until later, he said. There was plenty else to worry about in the meantime, he didn't say, but we knew.

Despite our constant worries, though, our baby did seem to be progressing. He was growing, gaining an ounce a day; his eyelashes came in, soft and downy; he was so strong, he rolled over for the first time at three weeks old. Every parent wants their child to be a prodigy, but we were sure of our son's particular genius. He was our hero; despite everything we had to do to him, the endless indignities of hospital life, and the many ways our plans for his entry into the world had gone off the tracks, he thrived. He was still breathing fast, taking about twice as many breaths as normal, but he would grow out of it, the nurses and doctors said. And he was lucky; he was not stricken by the respiratory infections and stomach blockages so common in such small infants. We were enthralled by our tiny warrior.

The first time he opened his eyes to watch us, his parents, talking, my heart changed form and function. It melted and reoriented itself around this little baby. The first time I held him in the NICU, he nestled like a tiny flightless bird on my chest. He was so tiny, so frail, but he also felt so marvelously real and solid after weeks of separation. I felt like I had too much oxygen in my lungs; I wanted to breathe in so much more than my chest could hold. From then on, I craved holding the baby, feeling his delicate skin against mine, his head resting contentedly above my heart.

But we had to measure our time with him carefully. He loved being held, even then, but the excitement wore him out and made him lose weight. So we limited ourselves: one hour, every other day. It only made me more eager for the moments when he nestled against my heart. It was the only time, in those long weeks, when I truly relaxed. I would close my eyes and feel him lifting and sinking gently with every breath I took. We were finally connected once again.

I imagine all new parents feel like imposters. I imagine they hold their new babies when they get home and terror strikes— *How am I supposed to care for this baby? I know nothing about newborns! Who approved this decision?!* But being a preemie parent adds a whole new layer of fear and doubt and vulnerability. Not only did we have to adjust to being brand-new parents, we also had to have a crash course in neonatal health.

One day, our baby's heart stopped beating. Neither Jack nor I was in the room, a fact for which I am simultaneously heartbroken and grateful. The nurses rushed over to check on him, and a moment later his heart began beating again. "Probably just the exertion of a bowel movement," the doctor explained when we arrived at his bedside only a few minutes later. "Sometimes it's hard to do more than one thing at a time."

The first time I saw my son choke, I was holding him. I felt him convulse a little, and then his face went blue and his eyes went wide. His mouth was working, but his chest was not rising or falling. He was staring at me, silently begging for me to do something. "Help!" I called out. "Please help me!" Two nurses rushed up and began sucking the vomit out of his nose and mouth with an aspirator. Mingled with my relief that they were there and he was fine, I felt searing guilt and confusion. What kind of mother was I to call for someone else to rescue him? Why couldn't I save him?

These feelings of fear and inadequacy sometimes paralyzed me, but more often they only made me more eager to be his mother every chance I got—even when it meant doing things I never expected to do. I jumped at every chance to change his diaper, take his temperature, even hold him down as the nurses drew blood, as hard as that was. I read the medical books and attended the doctors' rounds several times a week to ask questions. I was undertaking an education I never thought I'd need; one doctor joked that I was getting my nursing degree.

Soon, our education would be put to the test.

Our son's fast breathing wasn't slowing. By all other measures, he seemed to be developing fine, but still he took twice as many breaths as he should have; essentially, he was hyperventilating all of the time. The earliest possible date they'd said he could go home came and then went; he was still on oxygen, there was no way he could go home like this. His lungs should have been maturing, but if anything, his breathing seemed to be getting worse. And because he was taking so many breaths, he struggled to gain the weight he should have been putting on—even as we added caloric supplements to his breast milk. Everything exhausted him.

For the first five weeks of his NICU stay, we had surrendered to the medical staff. They knew what they were doing; they dealt with babies like this all of the time. We were the newcomers here. But as our son missed more milestones—going off oxygen, gaining more weight, transitioning to full-time bottle- and breastfeeding—we began asking more questions, trying to understand what we were missing. Had we misunderstood something? Was he still progressing as they expected? But the answers seemed to waver and scatter around us; we couldn't hold onto them, couldn't find any solidity. He went off oxygen, and then went back on. When we asked why—had he had trouble breathing overnight? Was this common?—we couldn't get a straight answer. Soon, we realized, our baby was flummoxing the professionals, too. No one was sure why he was breathing the way he was.

We could endure the long hospital stay; we could endure the procedures; we could endure leaving our baby in a sterile bed each night; we could endure the nurses and doctors caring for him instead of us. But this—this not knowing, this inability to help—this could break us. I felt powerless and guilty for putting our poor baby through all of this. I had to do better. I had to fight for him. Scenarios looped through my mind: Should I have him transferred to another, larger hospital? Should I show up in the NICU one day and demand he be discharged into my care against medical advice?

Jack and I called every medical friend we knew—a neurologist, a pulmonologist, even a veterinarian. *What should we do?* we asked, choking on tears, trying to hold back that breaking feeling. Our friends answered cautiously, not wanting to offer bad medical advice, cognizant of our doctors' boundaries. But their responses all came down to this: we had to trust that our son was getting the best care. If we didn't trust his medical team, we needed a new team.

Back at the hospital, the nurses began whispering to us. "He should be improving," one of them said.

"I think you should call the cardiologist," another said.

Yes. The cardiologist. It was a glimmer in the darkness; I seized upon it. We were due for a follow-up in one week, to check the hole in his heart. But the cardiologist was visiting another patient later that day, so she agreed to see my son, as well.

I held down his arms and legs, still so tiny, as she moved the ultrasound wand over his heart. She watched the blood, pulsing blue and red on the ancient ultrasound monitor. She scanned him carefully, methodically, and then she nodded and turned to me.

"The hole in his heart is definitely causing these breathing problems," she said, and I almost collapsed in tears. Not from fear over what this might mean. From joy. Finally, we had a reason, a diagnosis, a plan of care. The sweet relief of having answers, after weeks of fear and worry.

The hole existed when his heart formed, she explained; it was not caused by his prematurity. However, she said, his prematurity was likely exacerbating the heart condition. Perhaps if he had been born full-term, he wouldn't have struggled so; but that's how it was. He would need surgery to fix the hole, and probably soon, she said. And it wouldn't be a minor procedure; because of where the hole was positioned, he would need open-heart surgery. The surgeon would connect him to life support, crack open his sternum, pump him full of strangers' donated blood, and patch the hole, tiny but looming so large, with careful minuscule stitches.

Even though the idea of open-heart surgery weakened my knees, I was so happy I could have hugged her. We had a plan. This was movement. My baby was going to get better.

The cardiologist recommended transferring him to the larger regional hospital in order to monitor his heart every day and to discuss a plan for surgery. Once we decided to transfer him, everything happened quickly. The next day, we were riding in an ambulance. It was his first time outside. It was brief; after a twenty-minute ride, we wheeled him into the new hospital. And then things sped up even more. After five days, the team of doctors and specialists declared him to be in stable condition. We developed a plan for his care, setting appointments to follow up on the heart condition and evaluate him for surgery, and then they said we could go home.

/

Home. Home! For nine interminable weeks, it had been an impossible dream. From the day he was born, we had no idea whether he'd ever come home with us; the thought was so scary, so fraught, I'd pushed it out of my mind. Now the words hit me like a wave: *We could bring our baby home.*

We spent his discharge day in a flurry of activity. My husband left work early and went home to pick up the car seat, still in its box after all these weeks. Nurses performed the baby's hearing test and the car seat test, to make sure he could ride in the seat without exhibiting signs of distress. He passed both.

Now the hard part. Our son was still on a feeding tube, threaded down his nose and into his stomach, through which he also received several medications—including heart medicine, without which he might descend deeper into heart failure. I needed to learn how to operate the feeding machine we'd be taking home with us, and I needed to show the nurses that I could insert the feeding tube on my own when he inevitably pulled it out—something he did every few days.

I told the nurses at this new hospital it would be no problem; I'd been watching the other nurses maintain the tube for weeks; all they had to do was show me how to insert it. I pushed back my creeping unease, the little voice that said *But you've never actually done this before.* The truth was, I was scared of transferring his life into our hands. I was terrified of all that could go wrong on our watch. But I was also so, so ready to bring him home. I knew there was no limit on how far I would go, what I would do, for my son. Even if it hurt me. Even if he cried and protested. I would do it, I had to; there was no other way.

The nurse first demonstrated how to prepare everything. "Assemble all of the supplies first, because once you start, you'll want it all within reach," she said. We laid out a stethoscope, bandages, tape, a little bottle of sterile water, and the long thin feeding tube on his bed, arranged at his feet like gifts from exceedingly strange wise men. I cut up the tape and bandages, ready to plaster them over his cheek when the tube was in place. I dunked the tube in water to lubricate it, and then I began inserting it. Faster is better; faster, and then this would all be over. I pushed the tube up his nose, and he tipped his head back to cry. The nurse had warned me about this, and I was ready. I ignored his cry and I waited. As soon as he took a breath in the midst of his cries, I pushed the tube in, feeding it down his esophagus like a snake through the bathtub drain. I found the spot on the tube we'd marked, our stopping point, and placed the tape across his cheek, from nose to ear. He looked at me, a little stunned. I placed the stethoscope on the small rise below his ribs, at the top of his stomach, and with a syringe I pushed air into his belly and heard the sharp click of air hissing through the stethoscope earpieces. The tube was in place. I gratefully tore the stethoscope off.

"How was that?" I asked, suddenly exhausted, hating myself for everything I'd put my baby through.

"That was great!" the nurse said, looking relieved. I wondered if most parents were not so successful; if other parents heeded their babies' cries and stopped pushing. Not me.

With that final hurdle complete, we were done. Our baby was in the car seat, and then we were walking out of his hospital room and down the hall and out into the world.

We were the luckiest parents in the world.

And then we walked through our front door, and we were the most terrified parents in the world. We had fought so hard and for so long to bring him home. Now he was here, and he was so tiny, and he needed so much. What had we done?

The baby began stirring, and we looked at the clock: 11 p.m. Time for his next feeding. He was on a strict schedule, receiving two ounces of fortified breast milk every three hours. We set up the feeding machine, measured out the milk, and connected the machine to his feeding tube. Over the next forty-five minutes, the milk slowly dripped down into his stomach, and he dozed off again to the rocking of his new swing. When the meal was almost done, we measured out his meds with shaking hands. We were so careful to be precise; too much, and he could become violently ill; too little, and he would worsen. We lined up the syringes at the opening of the feeding tube and pushed the medicine through, and then we reconnected the line of milk.

As soon as the meal was finished, he woke up. It was almost midnight, and we'd spent the day running around, trying to prepare for his sudden arrival home. We were utterly exhausted. And now he was wide awake. I lifted him out of his swing and then laid him down on the couch. I knew we weren't supposed to move him after a meal, because it often triggered his reflux—projectile vomiting made worse, we would later learn, by his heart condition. But I was so tired, my foggy brain didn't compute what I was doing. Just as I remembered and reached out to scoop him back up, he vomited the entire feed—and his meds—all over the couch.

"Oh, baby, I'm so sorry!" I said, near tears, holding him against my chest, sticky face and all, as I made sure his nose and mouth were clear and tried to mop up the mess on the couch. "I should have known better!" I didn't know what to do—should I feed him again? I was too paranoid about the meds to give him another dose; I would wait until his next dose, in the morning, and hope he'd be okay until then. I had sudden visions of him worsening overnight, of us having to rush him back to the hospital, of the doctors and nurses wagging their heads and clucking *I-told-you-so*. Jack and I decided to wait and see if the baby got hungry—perhaps we'd bump up the next feed, which was supposed to be at 2 a.m., a little earlier. That's something about newborns I had never realized. Feeding every three hours meant that, after an hour-long feed, we only had two hours to rest.

And now the baby was even more awake.

We'd rushed around so much that day, and we'd been so taken

aback by his release, that we didn't even have his cradle ready for him. I set up a travel bassinet in our bedroom and laid him down. He looked so tiny lying there: just six pounds, six ounces. And he looked so naked without any wires or monitors. I was stricken with panic. What if something happened? What if he choked or his heart stopped beating again? With no monitors to watch over him, only these exhausted parents of his, how would he ever survive? Who were we to think we could care for this tiny baby who needed so much?

And who *was* this child in our home, wide awake and blinking up at us?

We thought we'd gotten to know him over the past nine weeks; we'd found him to be a sleepy, agreeable little guy. But we suddenly realized that, because his first NICU didn't have private rooms, we'd never slept there or cared for him this late at night. Now we were learning very quickly that we were the parents of a night owl. We were exhausted, frazzled, wondering if we'd made some terrible mistake, worried none of us would last through the night.

But we did. The baby finally relaxed against my chest and drifted off to sleep. At 2 a.m., and 5 a.m., and 8 a.m., and 11 a.m., we woke and fed the baby for an hour and then slipped back to sleep.

The days shimmered with sleep deprivation—falling asleep only to have the alarm go off in what seemed like a few minutes. But we were diligent in keeping the baby's feeding schedule. Part of me was still scared that the doctors would take him back to the hospital, so I settled into caring for him even more intently than before.

My biggest fear, aside from the wild terrors that sometimes kept me from dropping into immediate sleep at night, was whether the baby would choke again, like he had in the hospital. What would I do then, with no nurses rushing to my aid? I was afraid I would choke, too, that I would freeze and fail my baby in his greatest time of need. I felt keenly my failure, in the hospital, to step up and save my child. It plagued me when he came home.

But then it happened. After a feeding, the baby refluxed, and his breath didn't come. The vomit was stuck in his nose and mouth; he looked at me, eyes wide in breathless terror, lips turning blue. Just as I'd feared, panic flushed through me from head to toe. It felt like driving in a snowstorm and losing traction and sliding across the road. The loss of control, the blood-rush of panic, eyes fixed on the blind-white road ahead. I focused my entire being on getting back on track.

I grabbed his little rubber aspirator and quickly sucked the milk from his nose and mouth. *You can do this*, I told myself. I kept calm, even though it was a terrified calm. And when he took a ragged, grateful breath, I could finally breathe again, too. It had happened, and I had risen to overcome it. I could do this.

Soon, we settled into the rhythm of feeding and sleeping and changing diapers and onesies. We figured out his quirks, his personality, what worked and what didn't. We learned that he was not the kind of baby you could leave in a cradle to fall asleep on his own. We discovered that he was sleepy in the morning but he loved cuddling and playing with us at night. Even before he could control his movements or hold up his own head, he loved to dance. One day, when I sang to him as I was breastfeeding, he began humming, too, his bright eyes fixed happily on mine.

We followed his health extremely closely, consulting with cardiologists, pulmonologists, nephrologists, speech and physical therapists, and pediatricians. We read studies on the efficacy and side effects of his heart medications. When he was prescribed preventative antibiotics for a potential kidney condition, I was only reassured after I read dozens of studies and reports about superbugs and resistance, weighing the risks against the possibility of long-term kidney damage.

Once the baby was home from the hospital, we began seeing his cardiologist every two weeks. At each visit, we waited for the cardiologist to tell us what we needed to do. There was a certain freedom in relinquishing control—an inevitability in yielding to someone with more expertise.

But suddenly, we had the power.

"It's really up to you when he has the surgery," the cardiologist said after the baby had been home for a month. "He's doing so well at home, and he'll probably continue like this for the next few months."

Our surprise must have shown on our faces. After months of being told what to do—now we were in charge?

"You're the ones taking care of him. And you're doing a great job," she said. "He will need the surgery, so if you're ready to do it, let's do it. But if you want to wait a few months, we can do that, too."

She matter-of-factly described the procedure again: the life support, the cracked sternum, the blood transfusions, the hours of heavy anesthesia while a surgeon stitched our baby back together again. And then there were the risks: the possibilities of needing a pacemaker or contracting diseases from the trans-fusions. Death. The idea of losing our baby was always there, looming in the backs of our minds, but no one had talked so frankly about its likelihood yet.

I looked down at my son, his head bobbing with his quick inhalations, the feeding tube dangling from his taped cheek. I felt intensely weary. Not just for me and Jack, but for the baby. We were working around the clock to keep him alive, and we would have kept going forever if we needed too. But after months of medications and special care, our son wasn't improving. He spent most of his time recovering from breathing so fast. I wanted him to get chubby, to giggle until he lost his breath, to move and play. He was just surviving, not living. We needed to do the surgery at some point anyway; we might as well do it now.

As soon as we scheduled the surgery, I was stricken with guilt and dread. Was I just doing this to get out of his grueling care schedule? Was I putting my baby's life in danger simply because

I was tired? What if we were making things worse for him? Should I just try harder, do more, be more for him? I felt the enormous weight of his tiny body. I wanted to do what was best for him, but I wasn't sure what that was. When a situation is so complicated and fraught, there are no right and wrong decisions—only the decisions you make. In the moment, you may feel terror, you may feel hopelessly inept, you may want the real grown-ups to take over—but you can do it. Or so I kept telling myself.

Still, my anxiety heightened with each passing day. The week before the surgery, I was a mess. How could I bring this baby back to the hospital? What if he was there for another two months? What if he encountered complications? What if—my mind slipped and slid around the greatest horror, ever-present and yet unthinkable—he never came back home?

Every time I fed him, I watched him and I memorized his face, the way he dozed and then blinked back awake, the serious way he regarded my face. I was given a precious gift and I didn't know how long it would last, so I was trying to store up every treasure while I could.

The night before the surgery, my friend Rachel sent me an email. Her son had also had open-heart surgery for several conditions, including the one my baby was facing. It was a detailed, lengthy email about what to expect, from waiting during the surgery to navigating recovery. She talked about feeding tubes and oxygen intubation and medications, and as I read, I felt myself shrug a little: *Oh, we've been through that.* And the thought sent me bolt upright. We'd already been through so much. This was just another hurdle.

That night, I went to sleep at peace for the first time in months. We were doing the right thing. It was hard—sometimes the right thing is the hardest thing, too. But our son would be better for it. He would be fine; he would be better than fine.

The surgery? What can I say about the surgery except that it happened, and he came through it. That sense of peace stayed with me even as I wandered around the hospital aimlessly, numbly, all through the long hours waiting for news, and then, miraculously, the call that came through: He was fine, it was over, everything went great.

And when our baby boy woke up from the surgery, he looked up at us and grinned for the first time. He'd given us fleeting little smiles before, between labored breaths. But this was the first time he'd grinned, his whole face igniting with joy. My breath whooshed out of me. Seeing him already so happy, already improved—it was like my own heart slipped free from its anchor and soared. We had made the right decision. He was ready to start living.

The hospital pediatrician on call slipped into the room. She gave us an update, and then she did something none of the other doctors had done.

"How does he look to you?" she asked.

I took a moment, looking at this miracle baby. "He looks a little puffy still," I said. "He weighs much more than he did before the surgery, so he still has some fluids to pass. But his breathing is great." I paused, wondering if she wanted to hear the next part—if it mattered to her, or if she only wanted to know the clinical details. "He looked up at us and he smiled," I said, trying not to let the tears overwhelm me. "He's so—he's so *happy*."

"Wonderful," she said, beaming. "And your update is really helpful. I thought he looked a little puffy still, but you would know better than me—you're with him all the time. You're the experts."

Her words stayed with me. We were the experts on our baby. We may not always know the right thing to do in such a complicated case, but we would consult with the specialists and make the best decision we could. Yes, it was a huge responsibility. But yes, we could do this. We could care for this special baby.

After all, we were his parents.

/

Over the next few months and years, you'll make dozens of tiny and momentous decisions. You'll continue taking him to all of the specialists, but many more of the surprises will be joyous ones.

The first time he catches a cold, you'll wake up every hour to check his breathing. You'll let him wipe his nose on your shirt, and you'll feel like a real mom in that moment. You'll decide: Is he sick enough to take to the doctor? Or is he okay here at home? Either way, it'll be your decision, and you won't question it anymore.

You'll stop thinking about what bad luck having a preemie was. You will learn to abandon milestones, to stop measuring your baby against other children, because he is the person he is. Whenever he smiles up at you or laughs or lays his cheek against yours, you'll know you wouldn't have had it any other way because this child is perfect and brilliant and strong—and maybe you'll begin to realize that you are, too. Someday, you'll even stop thinking this was something you did, or something you deserved.

You'll keep blundering on, held together only by this intense sense of deep love. Somehow, you'll figure it out, step by shaky step.

And one day, when he looks up at you and says his first word, it will feel like the most natural name in the world. *Mama.*

Aspirations

BY JONATHAN FREEMAN-COPPADGE

The lights in the halls of the ninth floor of Boston Children's Hospital are dimmed, though it is only seven o'clock on a Tuesday in early June. Outside, the city is still choked with the last of the evening commute, the radiant heat from the concrete now warmer than the sun's diminished rays. Inside room 925, my husband, Darren, consults with a gastroenterologist and two nurses about our boy, four months old to the day, who is sleeping on the hospital-bed-cum-crib. The boy who, two hours earlier, cried himself through a long pang of hunger and whom we, at the doctor's behest, denied a meal. The boy who needs every calorie he can get to make up for his seven weeks' prematurity. The boy whose lungs have been taking in baby formula for the past four months. The boy whose tiny body will soon be pinned to the mattress by me and my husband as a nurse threads a plastic hose through his nostril, down his esophagus, into his stomach. When it is in, she will try to listen with a stethoscope as we blow air into the hose with a syringe. Gurgles means we've hit stomach acid—bull's-eye. Whooshing means we're in the lungs—go back to step one. But we will hear neither gurgles nor whooshing because the boy will rend the air with shrieks of terror, and so we will try another method—reverse the syringe. If fluid comes up, you're in the stomach. If not, go back to step one. It's important to be sure you've hit your target, because soon the nasogastric tube will be connected to a pump that will push one milliliter of formula every sixty seconds into either his stomach or his lungs. If he starts to turn purple, the nurse will tell us, we're in the wrong organ.

But all of this will happen hours from now. At this moment

I am standing in the hall outside room 925 calling Nancy, our social worker, because the doctor will not authorize this procedure until consent is given. And my husband and I cannot give consent because the boy in the bed is not yet our son.

I tell Nancy where we are and why. That the boy we call Langston but whose birth certificate reads Adonis has failed his barium swallow test. That we watched on the screen as a technician fired X-rays at his throat, that we saw without understanding the ghostly liquid pooling just above his epiglottis before slipping down the wrong tube. As the radiologist narrated Langston's incremental drowning, my skin went cold in the over-air-conditioned room. The last word I remember her speaking was "admit."

"They need to admit him," I tell Nancy. My voice is hoarse. I have already done my crying. "Probably three days. They want to give him a nasogastric tube for feeding while we consider options. The doctors won't do anything without consent from his legal guardians." I lean on the terms like crutches. Maybe if I speak like they do in TV shows, I too will make it to the end of the episode.

"Give the doctor my number," Nancy says. "And Jonathan, we should talk about what this means for you. Whether you want to move forward with the placement."

I want to dismiss her, to tell her that the boy in room 925 is ours, regardless of the fact that we are six months away from finalization.

"This could be a huge health concern," Nancy says into the silence, "and you need to consider whether you want to take on the risk."

"I'll talk to Darren," I say, my voice halting and rough. I will not cry again today; there is no time. We will need to drive the hour home, pack our bags, sort out dog care en route, alert the school administrators to my absence, and drive back into the city.

"I'll wait for the doctor's call," Nancy says, and we hang up.

Despite my promise, I will not raise Nancy's last question with Darren. I will not reify the idea of walking away from this boy, our boy, born in the very moments when we had been staring at our Valentine's Day dinner plates, grieving after four failed placements, while the nurses who would eventually become our first teachers in the art of parenthood were already performing their rituals over his tiny body.

/

We came into Langston's life at the end of his first month, a month he spent in the Pennsylvania hospital where he was born at thirty-three weeks and a hair over four pounds. His arrival was the end of an adoption process that began, for us, eighteen months earlier, a process full of work and preparation toward some indefinite end (Boy or girl? Tomorrow or next year? Newborn or one-year-old?). On the advice of our adoption agency, we told few people about our process so that, if things fell through, we wouldn't have to break the bad news to our entire social circle. We spent months preparing our nursery in secret, keeping the blinds closed so that my boarding school students would not look in and see a crib, fetching our packages from the mailroom after dark so that people would not see us lugging diapers, Boppy pillows, and Pack 'n Plays. When the agency called to say they had a potential match (as they did four times), I tried to hide any emotion as I instructed students in the intricacies of Shakespeare's procreation sonnets. When they called to say the match had fallen through (as they did three times), Darren and I would grieve in private and dry our tears before it was time to put the boys in our dormitory to bed. Some nights it felt like we would never be chosen.

When the final match came, only our closest friends knew where we were going. Even though the birth mother had already signed her release, we worried about unforeseen complications that might send us home empty-handed. Our arrival at the Pennsylvania hospital six hours away from our home outside of Boston was rich with dramatic tension, a sense of performing a great secret and also becoming audience members in our own life story where so much (the mother's decision, myriad adoption legalities, complicated hospital protocols) was out of our control. The new protagonist in our lives was a little boy whose lungs were too small to muster a full-throated cry. When he opened his translucent eyelids and looked at us, I felt the mantle of parenthood descend mysteriously and irrevocably upon me. The nurses became our directors, choreographing the timing and angle of our every move as we learned how to feed him, how to bathe him, how to monitor his oxygen saturation and his calorie intake. For all their graciousness with us, we were keenly aware of our own ignorance. What qualified us to take this fragile creature out of the care of the professionals? Did we seem as incompetent as we felt?

Four days after our arrival at the hospital, and four weeks after Langston's entry into the world, the hospital released us, and our enlarged family entered the world for the first time. We called Langston our little puppy when we put him into his car seat for the first time and he whimpered, our little frog when he tucked his limbs under him as he slept on our chests. We spent those first two weeks at my parents' house in Pennsylvania until adoption courts said we could leave the state. We felt the pressure of wanting to show my folks that we were up to this and to establish our role as Langston's primary caregivers. But we also benefited from their experience, from my mom's R.N. wisdom about his fluctuating body temperature to their offers to watch him while we took a walk.

We practiced everything we learned from the nurses, and improvised when Langston went off-book. The first time he lost color during a feeding felt like a nightmare where I couldn't speak or move fast enough to prevent a catastrophe. Suddenly

Darren was screaming at me that he was choking. Langston's change in color had been so gradual I had barely noticed it, and he gave no signs of distress. We cleared his airway quickly, but the clouds of fear and doubt began to gather on the horizon. Months later, after we settled back home in Massachusetts, we would recognize this as the first episode of silent aspiration that characterized his first four months of life—four months in which we experienced none of the connection that new parents gush about when they talk about feedings. Langston seemed distracted or lost in some inner world where we could not comfort him. He didn't cry or sputter, but it was clear he didn't relish the bottle.

"Something's wrong," Darren said on more than one occasion.

"Nothing's wrong," I said.

"Most babies don't cry like this all the time."

"What do you know about most babies?" I said. It was an unfair way to win an argument that should have never been an argument, but I was determined that Langston should be healthy, that his days in the hospital were over. He had been released to us after four traumatic weeks, and our job was to usher this fragile being into safety and health. What if we discovered something we weren't prepared to handle? What if we decided we *couldn't* be the parents Langston needed?

But as Langston's cries became more persistent and our frustration with our blasé pediatrician grew, I acquiesced to Darren's insistence that we get a second opinion. When a colleague offered to connect us with the gastroenterology department at Boston Children's, I took her up on it. When the gastroenterologist requested a barium swallow test to see if Langston was aspirating, I said yes because I knew it was the only thing that would put Darren at ease. When the test revealed that Langston was aspirating, and the radiologist told us that he would require immediate hospitalization, I cried as I held him in the waiting room. I cried for his pain and for my stubbornness, the willful ignorance that had put him in harm's way.

/

By the time we get back to BCH, almost ten hours after the barium swallow test, it is almost midnight. Langston is still asleep in the hospital bassinet, as are his roommates, a mother and daughter on the other side of the curtain partition. We will soon learn that the girl is twice Langston's age and half his weight. They arrived a few days earlier via medevac from their home in Alabama, where the father is arranging care for the twin brother. Darren and I try to settle in without waking anyone—folding the vinyl sleeper seat out into the room's diminishing square footage, taking our pajamas and toothbrushes to the hallway bathroom by the nurses' station, tuning out the ambient noise of the hospital even as nurses come in to check monitors.

When we wake, we hear the mother singing hymns to her daughter, songs familiar to me from my Evangelical upbringing, but her drawl as exotic in this city as our gay, interracial family might be in theirs. I wonder whether she sees our presence here, our inability to keep our boy healthy, as proof that gays make poor parents. I can hear my grandfather questioning whether we should really be bringing a child into a "homosexual household." I can hear my father warning me that our son would require nurturing that two men couldn't give him. I can hear Nancy questioning whether we are truly up to the challenge. And here we are, confirming everyone's doubts.

/

The next day, our shared room feels like a tunnel outside of space and time. Our roommates have the exterior portion of the room, so we have no sense of daylight. The girl's father arrives midmorning and we exchange cautious greetings. He looks like so many men I grew up around: jeans and flannel, a few tattoos peeking out from under rolled-up sleeves, a buzz haircut—the rural blue-collar uniform.

Darren and I mark time between doctors' rounds by shuffling down to the cafeteria and back, texting with friends and family who ask for more information than we have. I feel guilty in sharing the news, like I'm spoiling everyone's joy about our adoption. For exercise we pace the halls, pushing Langston's bassinet. Through open doors we can see other families—children without hair, without a limb, without speech; parents whose faces bear stripes of sleeplessness, helplessness. It feels like a communion of quiet love and sadness in sterile spaces. It feels like a vision of our future.

"Nancy called me," Darren says on one of our walks. "She asked whether we still wanted to pursue finalization."

"Mmhmm." I don't know how to say that she's already asked me that question. That I was too afraid to bring it up with him. That I'm scared by what we don't know about Langston's condition and whether we will be able to meet his needs. I can't imagine coming home without him, making calls to our family, explaining to all our friends and the students at the boarding school that the boy they helped us welcome is no longer ours. I swallow hard. "What did you say?"

"I told her the question hadn't occurred to me. But I said I would talk to you about it first."

We stop outside our room, where we can hear our roommates talking with their doctor.

"What do you think?" Darren asks.

I look down at Langston asleep in the bassinet. His hair, soft and straight since birth, has begun to curl upward, making him look a lifetime older than the boy we welcomed only three months earlier.

"I think this is our son, no matter what the paperwork says," I say, smoothing his curls down. "I can't imagine anything that would change that."

"Okay," Darren says, taking my hand.

When we finally get some information, it comes in a flood. Hospital employees whose names blur together come to educate us about how to operate the formula pump, how to secure the braces around Langston's arms to keep him from tearing the tube out of his nose, how to have our bills (now over $10,000) retroactively sent to MassHealth as a secondary insurer. Sometimes there are three of them in the room at the same time. When the nurse asks if we want to practice inserting an NG tube, we shake our heads.

"If it comes out, you'll have to take him to the pediatrician or to the ER," she says.

"That's okay," we say. "Both are five minutes from our apartment." I can't forget Langston's terrified screams when the first tube went in, or the nurse's less-than-foolproof guidelines about avoiding the lungs. Given the fact that he's been aspirating for the past four months under our care, I'm eager to leave the medical procedures to the professionals.

When the room finally clears, Darren turns to me blankly and asks, "Did you get all that?"

"I got the part about the pump, but I have no idea what we're supposed to do for the insurance, especially since he doesn't have a Social Security number yet."

Suddenly the father on the other side of the room speaks up. "It seems like it shouldn't be so hard just to take care of your kid, you know?"

I feel something tighten in me. Is his comment a critique or an attempt at solidarity?

"Like, how much red tape do you have to cut just to get your kid the care he needs?"

"Yeah," I say hesitantly. "It's a lot to take in."

"You guys are adopting him, right? And it's not even official yet, but you're the ones who have to figure out how to pay for it. Doesn't seem fair."

"It's not ideal," I concede. I'm caught between accepting his offer of sympathy and implying that I resent the demands put upon me as Langston's parent.

But his overture is the beginning of a bridge between our families. They tell us the saga of their twins, the doctors they've seen so far, the questions that loom, the ways their lives have had to change to accommodate their daughter's mysterious needs, the distances they have traveled to find answers. We tell them of Langston's adoption, of our days in the neonatal intensive care unit, and the ensuing months of fear and confusion. At the end, we sigh over each other's stories and extend generic expressions of hope, which are all we have to offer.

When my friend Danielle, an Episcopal priest who initiated us in the rite of shopping for baby supplies, comes to visit, I ask her if she'll take some extra time to pray with our Alabama roommates. "I don't think the multi-faith chaplain here really speaks their language," I tell her. I imagine how alone I'd feel if the hospital were in Birmingham instead of Boston. I want to make them feel at home in this strange place. Maybe they'll return home and tell their church how the New England gays supported them in their crisis.

Later, we bump into a few more families on our hallway circuit. We are learning that we are lucky to be here—lucky that a friend who had connections to the hospital could get us an appointment, lucky to live an hour away, lucky to have friends in the city who let us shower and feed us something besides hospital food. We exchange a nod with the other families, a kind observation about the beauty or bravery of our young ones, perhaps a tip on how to navigate the health care system's labyrinths. There is an understanding that here, with doctors and nurses and residents and roommates, the last thing anyone needs is another recounting of symptoms and procedures, another expression of sympathy, let alone any hint of competition between tragedies. The faces become familiar, and we feel we have entered into a secret society of parenting. I once thought parenting looked like the happy families I saw in parks, perhaps even those happily harried parents whose kitchen has become a war zone. I have never seen into spaces like the one we inhabit now, where the battle is not over whether our children *will* eat, but whether they *can* eat. Whether they will grow and thrive and do all those things we dreamed they would before they came into our lives. These parents exude a depth that rarely finds expression on the playground. There is an unspoken bond between us. We are all here for our own reasons, and that is enough to give and accept whatever grace we can afford.

/

On the day of our discharge, we are reserved but happy. Langston's diagnosis is uncertain but his prognosis is hopeful. The cause of his aspiration might be anatomical or neurological, but there is also a solid chance that it's a result of his prematurity. With a little more time we will either discover the cause or the problem will resolve itself. Whatever happens, we will soon be headed home, and that feels as victorious as the first time we left the NICU with him in our arms.

At lunchtime, we say goodbye to our roommates who are escaping the hospital for their first real meal. I don't know if we will keep in touch, but it doesn't feel necessary that we do. It is enough that we have been here together. We hook Langston up to the pump and begin a feeding while he naps. We head down to the cafeteria for our last hospital meal. As happy as we are to leave, we are nervous about what happens once we are away from the doctors and nurses upon whose expertise we have relied. Yes, we know how to run the formula pump and how to mix his medicines. But what don't we know that we don't know? What crucial precaution or red flag or essential paperwork are we going to miss without a team of experts to be responsible for us? And what about our new society of parents enduring similar struggles? How will we make it once we step back into a world that still asks "How's it going?" and expects you to answer "Fine"?

After lunch we ride the elevator back to the ninth floor in what feels like a valedictory lap. We have already checked out, so it is simply a matter of collecting our bags and getting the car.

"I'll grab the bags and meet you and Langston at the front of the hospital with the car," I tell Darren.

But when we get back to the room, Langston is already awake, sitting in a puddle of formula, arm braces hanging loosely from his elbows, the NG tube conspicuously absent from his nose. He looks at us with as much pride as a four-month-old can muster.

"Well," Darren laughs, "I guess we're learning how to insert an NG tube!"

The process is awful and survivable, which is exactly how we'll describe the next few months as we develop new rhythms and routines for Langston's care. The nurse's warning about him turning purple will haunt us for each of the thirteen NG tubes Darren and I will insert over the next six weeks, a process that will only get harder as Langston begins to understand and resist what is happening to him. Most of the insertions will happen at 6:00 a.m., after he's had a night to break free of the braces and work the tube out of his nose. As terrible as each reinsertion is, I'm glad we don't have to make thirteen early-morning trips to the ER.

/

Four years later, I still worry that I'm not equipped to give my son what he needs. But I'm also learning to lean on the community of those who fight for their kids and for each other. I still fear that my son's needs are an indictment of my own inadequacies. But I'm also learning how to ask for the expertise and resources he deserves. I'm still overly self-conscious about what people think of me and my family, but I am coming to embrace the fellowship of families held together by the fierce love we have for our children, one that is stronger than any geographical or theological bond.

When I think back on the parent I used to be, the one who thought parenthood was comprised of park playdates and Insta-worthy mealtime messes, I hardly recognize myself. It feels like Darren and I are earning our stripes, the same ones I saw on those other parents in the hospital. I used to fear I might become them. These days, that sounds like a worthy aspiration.

Simon's Story

BY MEGAN WALKER

"I think it's time to call your husband," my labor and delivery nurse said anxiously, watching me writhe through another contraction.

"I'm fine. We're fine. This is just a scare." I tried straightening myself from a curled position, crinkling the mattress cover beneath me.

"Fine" was my doctor-husband's favorite word.

"Everything will be fine," he'd say. Over a skinned knee, a broken heart, a hole in our window or roof. "It'll all turn out okay."

I usually responded with a scowl or a slap on his shoulder and a lecture on how unfeeling or insensitive he was when it came to serious problems. But as I lay alone in that hospital bed, he was fifteen minutes away with our other two children. I willed his words to be true, hearing his voice in my head. *We will be fine. My baby, my son, will be fine.*

Having been admitted into the antepartum unit at twenty-four weeks, I knew the risks of a premature baby, knew the statistics of survival at every gestational period, and none of it was positive. Reading story after story of amazing miracles and tragic deaths did nothing to appease my worried heart, but still I read them.

Which would be my son? The miracle story, the one who surpassed every challenge, who overcame the odds, who was given that special title—*The One Who Came Home.* Or the tragedy? With the mother who, despite everything she prayed and ached for, would've given her own heart, lungs, every drop of blood within her, held her child as he took his final breath.

Left with only a picture and tiny memories to speak for a huge little life.

As I finally made that phone call, crying to my husband that, the time had actually come at twenty-six weeks and four days' gestation, I prayed for the millionth time for a miracle. *Please, God, let him stay. Please don't take my son away. Please give him good lungs, a good, strong heart, and give me more time.*

/

Ted burst through the door to my room, a look of panic in his eyes, but the most tender, kind sound to his voice. He held me, breathing through each contraction with me, while watching the Doppler for any indication that our baby's heart grew tired. Within minutes of my husband's arrival, the first deceleration lit up the screen. A nurse ran in, studying the printed paper that showed the dip in heart rate.

"He's getting tired," she said, calling in a doctor.

As brilliant as doctors and health care providers are, when you've interacted with them regularly you can read the signs all over their faces when something is wrong. There is something in their smiles. A light that does not reach their eyes. A sympathetic wrinkling of their foreheads. I knew as soon as I saw our doctor that our time was up, and it took my breath away.

"How are you feeling?" she asked, motioning to several other nurses to join our room. "I hear your little man isn't cooperating today."

A false chuckle, and Ted and I shared a knowing look. She was trying to lighten the mood, trying to give us that brief moment of positivity before the worst news hit.

Simon was not the kind of baby to wait around for pleasantries, though. He was classy, regal, no-nonsense, and he wasn't going to let this doctor dawdle. His heart rate dipped lower, stopping for a moment, before slowly creeping back up.

"It's time. We need to get him out now," the doctor said suddenly, and the rest was a blur.

One nurse took my wedding ring, and then Ted's. Another brought in a bed to transfer me onto, and I vaguely remember getting a new robe. Questions came from every angle. "You'll be getting a spinal, are you allergic to anything?" "Are you aware of the risks?" "Do you want your husband by your side?"

A surgeon met us at the foot of the bed, walking in front of us while calmly spouting off information about the surgery and what to expect. Did he honestly think I was listening to him? I felt like I was having a seizure for the shock waving through my body. *This cannot be happening. This isn't happening. How did I get here?*

I'd always known I wanted to be a mother. It felt natural, easy. My favorite job was babysitting, and my chosen profession, a kindergarten teacher, came from the knowledge that I would one day raise a houseful of my own children. My daughter, Sophie, came first, followed two years later by Owen. Simon was set to be exactly two years after Owen. A perfect trio.

But life had thrown me a curveball. God showed me once again that making plans, taking control of what I thought would be perfect, was not always going to be pain-free.

Ted was getting dressed in scrubs, and I was alone in the operating room. An amazing nurse I'd first met two weeks prior, on admittance into the hospital, was robed and hidden behind a mask. Still, I recognized her, and I will always remember the instant comfort of her eyes. She'd heard I was heading to the OR, and she stayed by my side, holding my hand the whole time, while Ted watched our medical team. He wore our camera around his neck.

A spinal. An oxygen mask. A cut and a tug hidden behind a curtain and Simon was out, but my ears waited in vain for his cries. Only silence, the rustling of panicked hands, and the beeping of machines filled the space.

I knew that without a breathing tube, Simon wouldn't make it. My angel nurse craned her neck to update me on the intubation process. "They failed. They're trying again. No, no, it's okay. They're trying again, it's not over. I'm trying to see. They're all so crowded, everyone is trying. It's still not going in."

Moments felt like hours. I couldn't breathe, but the oxygen still poured into my nose. *He'll live. Everything will be fine. Fine. Fine. Fine.*

This cannot happen to me. I cannot lose my baby.

"They've got it. It's in." My nurse squeezed my hand.

"Is he breathing?"

"He's okay."

I finally took a breath. All pain subsided. I felt the tugs, the pulls of the doctors cauterizing vessels in my body, sewing up a Simon-sized hole. But he was out. And he lived. And for now, that was good enough.

/

When he was stable, they rolled the baby's incubator over to me. I'd never seen such a box—clear and all-encompassing. I took off my oxygen mask and struggled to lift my head, but still couldn't see him fully. He was a tiny human covered in clear plastic; they told me it insulated him.

My entire body was overcome. It was painful to experience both intense joy and incredible sorrow at the same time. The statistics still bit at me. I knew the odds. But he was alive. That was the first step.

"Hi, Sparkle," I called, using the name lovingly chosen much earlier by my four-year-old daughter, Sophie. It would still be days before I chose his name: Simon. "Momma's here," I told him.

Instantly, his two tiny legs and tiny arms the size of my pinky finger shot up into the air.

"He knows his Momma," a man laughed. And I joined in through my tears.

Despite it all, my heart overflowed with love. For Simon. For my family. For a Father in Heaven who had not forsaken me.

I watched them wheel my tiny son away to the neonatal intensive care unit.

/

I am grateful for tough nurses.

Simon's first NICU nurse was more than tough. She was borderline pushy, but I admired her for it.

"You ready to change his diaper?" she asked on day two.

"Me?" My eyes grew wide. Simon was just over a pound. Surely I would break him. Who was I to change my own son's diaper? Isn't that what the nurses were for?

"Yes, you. You're his mom, aren't you?" She cast me a pointed glance as she gathered things for Simon's first care of the day.

"You're going to help me, right?" I looked at Simon in his incubator. He was tiny, and though his breathing tube was removed and he now breathed with nasal-prong oxygen through a CPAP machine, his fragility terrified me.

"Have you never changed a diaper before?"

I knew she was goading me, but I did not find it very funny at the time. I'd changed two children's worth of diapers and then some. But I'd never changed a tiny diaper. A diaper the size of my palm.

"It's the same here. Just watch his cords, and you'll be fine."

"But what if I'm not? What if I wipe too hard, or poke him, or touch something that instantly kills him?"

Any of those options seemed highly plausible. But my nurse only stared at me, hands on her hips, waiting.

That first diaper change was terrifying, to say the least. I lifted his legs like they were air. *Is this normal?* I thought. *Of course it isn't. My baby is the size of a Barbie doll.* He grunted and squeaked in displeasure as I wiped his nonexistent, flat little bum, and my heart filled. Motherhood overwhelmed me. Sophie and Owen had both hated diaper changes as babies, and now I could add Simon to that list.

"You're fine," I coddled him, chiding myself for the words my husband so often spoke. And yet they'd rung true for us so far. "Momma's right here, Si."

That nurse was also the one who pushed me to hold my tiny son later that day. Those same fears, same worries paralyzed me and made me forget my own worth. Who was I compared to a nurse whose experience surpassed my age? Or a doctor who knew how to intubate in an emergency? Besides, my body had yet to heal. I still struggled to stand for longer than five minutes, still took painkillers to ward off the pain of my incision. But one thing you learn about the NICU early on is that time is not guaranteed. A roller coaster is what they call the journey, and there is no greater way to describe it.

So I settled into my blue rocking chair, padded with pillows behind my back, my head, and under each arm. The tiniest little body wrapped in a dozen cords was placed on my chest and nestled safely into my shirt. He fit perfectly between my breasts, warm and perfect and so impossibly small.

There are not words to describe the first time a mother holds her child. The feelings of joy, pride, pure love, and relief. I felt it all in that moment, and then some. But this time there was a nagging voice that clawed in, full of logic. Those statistics and risk factors I'd read about and discussed with doctors and nurses over and over again. Necrotizing enterocolitis (NEC). Brain bleeds. Patent ductus arteriosus (PDA). Lung disease. Failure to thrive.

That couldn't happen to my son. Could it?

As his tiny hand of barely formed pink fingers wrapped around mine, I cried and laughed and cried. *Everything would be fine.* It had to be.

/

His squeaks became my morning call. I'd walk into the room each morning and even if he was in a deep sleep, I'd say, "Good morning, Si!" And before he'd even open his tiny eyes, he'd squeal for me to pick him up.

At first, I needed help to hold him. And my nurses were happy to oblige. It became a time for me to get to know "my people." As we changed his diapers, took his blood pressure and temperature, I'd ask about their lives, their families, their hobbies. We'd chat about everything from crabby neighbors to life plans, and these nurses and doctors became my best friends.

On rare occasions, I'd get a nurse I did not know well, and I'd stalk the hallway in anticipation of her help. *I know it only takes you two minutes to help me,* I'd think. *So I will stand here and make you uncomfortable until you do.* Most of the time they assisted me quickly. When they finished their current task, they'd grab a buddy nurse and help me get Si out of bed. I soon learned that to get what I wanted sometimes required courage and confidence, both of which I initially lacked. But each time I'd remind myself, *This is my son. He needs me. This is his journey and I'm not going anywhere.*

As moms, we have to be brave for our children. For Sophie, that meant smiling as I bandaged up a scraped knee or going on the pirate ship ride at Six Flags. For Owen, it was stopping up a bloody nose in the middle of the night and defending his wild behavior amidst a grocery store full of stares.

But for Simon, it meant standing up for our time together. I had to find my voice. That didn't mean being angry or rude, or expecting our great nurses and doctors to drop everything at our beck and call. It meant speaking up for myself and for my son. It meant going the extra mile to make my intentions and desires known, even if said intentions changed ten times in ten minutes.

Time flies in the NICU, and you'll never get it back. So make it your own. The greatest regrets I have are about the times I stayed silent. You can never go back and do more. It's what you did say, when you did hold him, or change his diapers, or try. Those are the times you'll look back on with gratitude, no matter how afraid you felt at the time.

/

Simon grew to two pounds, then three. The dimples in his chin and cheeks grew more pronounced, and he lost all of his preemie hair. Before long, I'd read aloud four Harry Potter books to him. Everyone knew my Voldemort impression. And at least half the team had seen my breasts. I pumped, pumped, pumped. Breast milk was something only I could give especially for him, and so I chose to do that. I became good friends with the lead breastfeeding advocate, who visited me regularly. She'd see me in the halls and poke fun at me for wearing comfortable clothes that looked like pajamas. I'd troll back about how expensive my leggings were and she'd cackle as we passed each other. She invited me to breastfeeding luncheons, and although I never wanted to leave Simon, sometimes I joined her. I made friends eating lunch in a small room right outside the NICU doors. The NICU became real. Room 505 was now my second home. Two of my children lived at one home, and my third child lived at the other. Neither was satisfying without the other. I lived in a constant state of guilt no matter where I was, but I tried. I made a village within the NICU. Some friends went home with their babies. Others didn't.

I remember passing a girl in the hallway on my way out one day. She was bawling, face red, cheeks drenched in tears, while she relayed news to her mother and family members. I heard tidbits as I waited for the elevator to drive home to Sophie and Owen. Something about her son's heart and not knowing how much longer they had.

A few days later, I saw her in a room outside the NICU and introduced myself. She was so kind, and we became instant friends. Over the course of a quick lunch, we discovered that not only did our sons share the same name and close birthdates, but our husbands were both in training for medical degrees. We exchanged information and saw each other many times at lunch and in the halls. Then one day, several months later, she and her husband passed me eating dinner in that same room. She told me her Simon was dying, and he would not recover. I held her tightly through her tears and told her how sorry I was. We stayed in touch during their last week together. I brought her a necklace and texted her to tell her how much I was thinking of her and her sweet Simon. The NICU felt different the day he left it. The line between Heaven and Earth so thin. Death became real, tangible, and crueler than I'd ever known it. And for our family, it became more of a possibility than we'd ever realized. Not everyone leaves the NICU with the miracle of healing. We cherished every moment forward after that day.

/

Three months passed in Room 505. It smelled like sanitizer and plastic, mixed with dirty feet from Simon's pulse oximeter. I soaked it up. I took the hospital-grade sanitizing wipes and followed the example of our nurses, gloving my hands and wiping down every surface I could see twice a day. I organized his little box and then his crib as he grew. Sophie and Owen colored pictures that I hung on his walls next to our family portraits. I hung a sign over his crib that read, "Simon, king of the NICU." And eventually it was joined by a bigger sign with Simon's likes and dislikes and a "what to do if's" list. A nurse told me that a past patient listened to a recording of his mom's voice when she was away at work, so I promptly went to Walmart and bought a recorder, documenting thirty minutes of reading aloud my kids' favorite books followed by singing our favorite songs. At first I was mortified to leave the device with my nurses. I am not someone who easily gets embarrassed, but I also did not believe anyone wanted to hear my voice read *Curious George* or sing church songs all night.

But Simon loved it. When I'd call before I closed my eyes each night, his nurses would often tell me that the recorder had calmed him to sleep. So we knew when the recorder wasn't helping, something was wrong.

Those calls were the worst.

"He's not settling down, we just wanted to make you aware."

"Should I come in? I'm going to come in," I'd say, half out of bed.

"No, no. You rest. We'll call you if any of his settings change, but we wanted to make you aware."

Evenings like that were usually followed by a bad day.

Simon had many bad days. I'd love to say our time in the NICU was filled with laughter and sweet newborn memories, but the truth is a lot of it was impossibly hard.

I was not always brave.

After a month or so of his oxygen levels worsening, Simon had a really bad day. Over time, Simon's doctors tracked small cysts on his lungs as they grew larger and then spread, eradicating healthy lung tissue. These "blebs" are common in preemie babies who require so much oxygen support, but the hope was that his lungs would improve or at least stop the disease from progressing.

As I held him that morning, his little body—now the size of a normal newborn baby's—pulled and tugged forcefully as he breathed. I took in steady breaths, wishing my lungs could do the work for his, but still his body struggled for a full breath.

Soon, our doctor came in and ordered an echocardiogram, or images of the heart, to rule out holes.

The diagnosis: severe pulmonary hypertension. Our next step

was reintubation. Back to square one. Without more support, Simon's heart would fail or arrest at any moment. But if we could give him time, perhaps his lung tissue would grow. Perhaps his body would heal. Our new goal would be to extubate and then keep him improving.

Ted ran over from the hospital where he worked, which was luckily connected to Simon's, and he and I gave Simon kisses as his nurses readied his room for the procedure.

That was the last time I heard Simon's voice.

Intubation was successful, and within days his pulmonary pressures improved, meaning his heart issues were indeed secondary to his lung disease.

After a visit from the Easter bunny and another month of no improvement, we met with an amazing team of pulmonary specialists to determine a plan for Simon's future.

Care conferences seemed useless and unhelpful each time our team brought us in to make goals. I remember sitting across the table from this obviously smart man, dressed sharply in round spectacles and a crisp bow tie. He smiled and joked as though life was just grand, and then told us that our son's lung disease was like none he had ever seen. That it wasn't improving. That it may never improve. And that our only option besides ending care was a tracheostomy that would likely last many years, if not his lifetime. The tube would bring air through an opening just above his collarbone, below his tiny vocal cords, and down into his overworked lungs.

I love that doctor. I always will. I know there is no easy way to tell parents such difficult realities. I am grateful men like him dedicate their lives to the care and healing of children. I just wish there were a painless way to hear bad news.

/

We chose the tracheostomy. I'd seen other babies with them, and though I was afraid, something told me things would be all right. A feeling in my heart confirmed that we were making the right decision.

A strange dynamic of the children's hospital is that you have no idea what other people are going through, but you could guess that it's really bad and be right nine times out of ten. Downstairs in the surgical waiting room, I sat next to complete strangers while I waited to hear if Simon survived surgery that afternoon. No one could have possibly guessed why we were there or what news we awaited. To an outsider, that room must've looked like any other waiting room in a clinic. We were normal, everyday people.

It reminded me of the time we were asked to leave the NICU temporarily because our neighbor's baby was getting surgery. I hardly knew this new family, but I knew that their son was on ECMO (extracorporeal life support) and things were not looking good. Because we could not be in the NICU during the bedside surgery, Ted and I took the opportunity to see the new *Beauty and the Beast* movie with Sophie and Owen at our local theater. My stomach was sick the whole time. I should be with my son. I should not be in a germ-ridden movie theater that could infect me and keep me away from his bedside even longer. But how wonderful it was to be with Sophie and Owen. We never had enough time together. They couldn't stay in the hospital for too long, because it could not contain their energy and I feared for Simon's cords and devices—not to mention the germs they surely carried on their little fingers and breaths.

As I sat in my fully sanitized theater seat, munching mindlessly on more popcorn than I'd had in months, I tried so hard to focus on the movie despite checking my phone a million times for messages. I remember being way too emotional during the Beast's song. From the outside, I probably seemed entirely unstable. And I was. But my burdens, my fears, my pain were all invisible to a stranger.

/

Simon lived through his own surgery, and he flourished with his trach for several weeks. His eyes peeked drunkenly at mine when I saw him trached for the first time. The corners of his lips twitched, and I knew we'd done the right thing. Even if it meant years of night nurses and special equipment and unbearable fear. Everything would be fine as long as I had Simon.

Month four was off to a great start. I'd never been happier. I had my Simon back! Therapies we could not previously do because of Simon's tube now helped to loosen his muscles and comfort him. He got a baby swing, which he loved, and he renewed his obsession with his pacifier. We even got to sit him up in a chair on one particularly good day. He did not last long sitting up, but it was such a huge deal to me. My Simon, sitting up! You couldn't have wiped the smile off of my face that day. Sophie and Owen even came in and rubbed his feet and legs. I was in heaven.

The trach was a learning curve for me, just as everything was. But after changing his trach ties a few times, I became more comfortable touching and adjusting them, and even recognizing smells associated with infection. I caught one infection before my nurses did.

Unfortunately, the good days were only part of the roller coaster. One day, Simon's respirations were struggling. His nurse and I decided to do a trach change. Because I'd been rocking his trach changes in days previous, I took charge. To this day, I do not know what exactly went wrong, but somehow Simon's trach twisted and he was not receiving the oxygen he needed for a few seconds. His nurse and I quickly discovered the problem and adjusted the trach, but Simon was not recovering. His face began to turn blue, and he was still. We sounded an alarm and within seconds, nurses and doctors both familiar and unfamiliar flew into our room, taking over Simon's care. I fell into the background, too stunned to speak. Too scared to move. What had I done? Why had I even tried to care for my son? Who was I to think I could do this? And the question I asked so often, so earnestly: Why was this happening to us?

I wanted to race from the room. I wanted to hide in a stairwell and cry until I could not feel this pain anymore. It ripped my heart and tore every bit of me into pieces. It was a physical pain, like a thousand tons of weight crushing me until I could not breathe. But motherhood anchored me to my chair. No matter how hard, how painful, or how terrifying the journey, it was Simon's. And I would share it with him.

Many other moments like that followed later. I watched him struggle to breathe for no apparent reason, turning blue, while frantic nurses and doctors tried to determine better respiratory settings to soothe him without hurting him. It is not in human nature to be comfortable with watching your child suffer this way, and as a result I have PTSD that rears its ugly head all too often, even now. Nothing could have prevented it, but the best medicine has been talking to people who have experienced similar complications with their children. You truly cannot comprehend the feelings and the shock until you've lived them. Even some of our amazing staff did not know how to treat me in moments of despair. Having a sick patient is different; witnessing a tragedy as a friend or neighbor is different. A grieving mom doesn't need you to know her pain. She just needs your compassion and love.

/

Then Simon had four bad days in a row. We tried everything. Different trachs, new sizes, and every different setting both the doctors and I could find, but still his breathing worsened. I considered transferring Simon to another hospital that specialized in bronchopulmonary dysplasia. I spoke with our doctors, and they agreed to try the same settings that hospital would have used. I monitored the changes consistently, and I knew what did and didn't work for Simon. One night, when Simon was not feeling well, a nurse practitioner and an overnight fellow struggled to find the appropriate settings to help him breathe. His saturations were falling, and things were not looking good.

The nurse practitioner turned to me and said, "There is nothing more we can do."

I remember thinking, *Is that what you are seriously saying to me right now? How am I supposed to respond to that?* I wanted our daytime doctor, I wanted the fellow I trusted the most and the nurses who knew my Simon best. Having no time to think, all I could say was "No."

I explained what had worked in days past, which settings the specialized hospital called for, and that at the very least we would attempt them before we could say with surety that there was nothing left to do.

Those settings worked.

Because of my voice, my adamance, my insistence, we got more time with our son. I saw his eyes one more time. I held him, kissed his head, his nose, his cheeks once more while he was awake. If there is one thing I do not regret, it was being informed to the point of arrogance. It was knowing the inside and outside of Room 505 and its workings. To any NICU mom, I would say, "Be a Momma bear. Be your child's advocate. Have courage. Speak. Stand for the child you've been given. It's okay to feel inadequate. What you are is enough. You don't need to be a doctor, a nurse, a professional. You be Mom. Listen to your gut, your feelings, your intuition. You are the one constant. And no one can replace you. Period."

But Simon's lungs grew stiff and weak. Days later, he would require 100 percent oxygen support indefinitely. We tried everything. Our doctors were devastated and frustrated that what should be working did not help. He was not sick by infection. His lungs were failing. We watched and waited in vain for Simon to wake up. To start breathing on his own. To come back to us.

In those final days, my body lived numbly while my mind and spirit tried to make sense of what we were witnessing. I'd seen babies of different sizes defy odds, overcome ECMO support, battle heart, brain, lung, and countless other surgeries and complications. Why was my son dying, while those children lived?

I sat at his bedside punishing myself for everything I'd done wrong. I should have spent more time at the hospital. I should've brought the kids to see him more. I should've forced my husband to trade places with me so that he could hold Simon longer. I should've let my daughter hold him. I shouldn't have been so scared. But then again, had I not been this germaphobic isolated mom, what else might have happened to Simon? Would he have died from some illness earlier? I can't know.

More cords, more lines, more medicines that numbed Simon's pain and paralyzed him. There was no explanation for how I found strength in my weakest moment, other than my firm knowledge that we have a loving God, a Father in Heaven, who loved and supported me. He did not take away my sorrow. He did not heal my son. But He also did not leave me comfortless.

Standing there beside Simon as machines breathed for him, I thought back to the day of my c-section. Suddenly, none of that seemed so bad. Hemorrhaging for ten weeks, then lying in the antepartum ward for more than two weeks. An emergency procedure followed by five of the hardest, yet happiest, months of my life. With Simon. I could fill pages with how brightly his eyes would gaze into mine, how we'd stare at each other for an hour. His fingers curling around my thumb. How it felt to kiss his chunky cheeks. After every bath, I'd brush his hair. His eyes would grow sleepy, and we'd rock and sing. Then I'd wrap him up in his blankie nice and tight, and sneak him into his crib. Some nights, he'd open his eyes just enough to make me stay. And we'd watch each other until his eyelids grew too heavy.

His final days were the hardest days of my life. I often tell my friends and family that there will be no harder days than what I have already lived through. The words spoken to us, the impossible choices we made, and what we saw ... there is no reason to put any of it into words, because it is unfathomable to anyone who has not lived through the loss of a child. Before Simon, I had no idea such physical suffering from heartache was possible for a human being. I wanted to die from the pain. I thought I was dying. I wished I was. Nothing can prepare you for it. You cannot imagine it. Don't try. And be grateful that you do not understand it.

I reached out to a few moms who could understand, who had lost their children before me. Their advice was priceless. One mom told me, "Cherish your time." It is morbid at first to think about cherishing those last moments. But I am so grateful that this friend gave me the encouragement to walk with my son as his heart slowed its beating. I held him as I never had been able to before. It was misery and despair in its most acute form, but it was also so very sacred to have a brief moment of what should have been. My perfect son, free of cords in my arms, as I whispered my love to him under the sunshine and shade of the trees. I know with a surety that we were surrounded by angels in that garden above the hospital. I felt the presence of Heaven. It is unexplainable. Amidst insurmountable pain, there was hope, love, comfort, gratitude. My heart, though broken, was encompassed by love.

This same friend encouraged me to hold on to how I felt in the moment. She said there would be moments when I would feel peace or comfort, when I would know that what was happening needed to happen. Holding on to those feelings or experiences, even writing them down, would bring immense relief in my life to come. I can say for a surety that my moments came. They are the only things that keep me living some days.

Oh, how I miss my Simon. How I long to forget that final morning, to imagine that he still lives in our NICU. That he waits for me in our little room even now.

/

We have treasured our time at his gravesite. Before, I couldn't understand why loved ones flocked to the graves of their deceased. "It's just a body," I'd think, knowing that the spirit lives on in Heaven. Now as we drive that gravel path to the sweet tree that shades Si's grave, I imagine him there, grown up and sitting against the tree trunk, waiting for me.

I feel Simon in my life every day. I see him in my dreams, I imagine him in my thoughts, I wonder what he is doing and if he misses me. I talk to him, and I feel impressions of his personality so often. Heaven must be near. It must be closer than we think. Every time we visit Simon's grave, my kids and I sing three songs. If the sun is already shining, it shines brighter. But even on the cloudiest day, when we sing, sunshine splits the sky. And I know it's Simon, shining just for me.

An Aunt in Your Corner

BY MARIA RAMOS-CHERTOK

Meeting my niece Sonia for the first time had much in common with the excitement that characterizes other firsts: first date, first job interview, first kiss. But it also felt different from those anticipated milestones, as this experience was filled with more paralyzing fear and dread than anything else I had ever done. My sister had prematurely given birth to twins: Sonia, weighing in at two pounds, two ounces, and Kai, who at fourteen ounces was struggling to survive. They had been in the neonatal intensive care unit in a New York hospital for two months by the time I flew from California to meet them.

Prior to my arrival, my sister and I talked on the phone whenever it worked for her schedule. We texted nonstop. I let her know she could call me any time, night or day. Uncharacteristically, I left my cell phone turned on and placed it next my bed each night. I had to be very intentional about putting her needs before my own desire to know everything that was happening each day. She told me how almost everyone she interacted with repeated that they "were praying for the babies." Hearing that started to feel burdensome to her. Was G-D involved in the decision to keep her children alive? If one didn't make it, did that mean G-D had made that decision? If so, how might she stay in a relationship with such a force? These profound questions were the murky backdrop against a landscape of unknown outcomes and deeply held desires for both of her children to survive and thrive. I knew that our conversations were a time for her to decompress and work through many of these thoughts and fears.

When I arrived at the hospital, I embraced new terminology: "NICU" was now a part of every other sentence. Hand sanitizer and hypervigilance about germs quickly became paramount in my mind.

In person, I had no idea how I would offer support to my sister and her husband. I was concerned that my presence, while welcome, could also be a burden. I feared they would feel the pressure to attend to me in some way, and that was the last thing I wanted. I knew how to help parents with newborns and I was comfortable holding, rocking, feeding, and changing diapers, but this visit would allow for none of that.

The day of my arrival coincided with an enormous decision they had to make about whether to remove all of the life-sustaining mechanisms keeping their son alive. My insides tremored. This would certainly be a day when they needed my support, yet I felt empty trying to conjure up what emotional sustenance I might offer. It was like the self I knew left my body, and only an outline of a person remained—a person who felt like an alien walking through an unfamiliar landscape: new equipment, new procedures, new people who knew way more than I did about how to deliver what was needed. Every few minutes, a hospital worker came in to perform a procedure, assess a situation, offer guidance, ask a question, or monitor progress. I was overwhelmed after being there for five hours. My sister, her husband, and their newborns had been living in this flurry of activity for two months.

Getting phone updates is one thing, but being in the room made me feel like my life had started over in the middle of a drama that I was a part of but hadn't been given a discernable role in. I felt like I was dreaming, and I wanted to wake up so I could return to the pre-dream state where the bad thing never happened. But the bad thing was very real, and it was happening during my first day in the NICU. The searing pain only deepened as conversations progressed about the end of life for my nephew Kai.

Knowing that Kai's parents needed to focus on him, I steered my energy to his sister, Sonia.

When I saw my niece for the first time, I was captivated by her tininess. I had no idea fingers and toes and lips could come in size extra, extra small. Yet she was perfect in every way. "Talk to her," someone said, so I did. I told her about how much I'd been looking forward to meeting her. I told her about going to the beach and eating ice cream, about Pablo Neruda's poetry; I promised I'd buy her one of his books. I told her about her cousins, my two sons, and how they wished they could be here with me. I told her about California, about the Golden Gate Bridge; I told her that one day she would visit me there, and about the fun we'd have. I described her uncle Keith, or "Tio Keith." I told her that life was waiting for her, and that we had lots and lots to do together. I talked and talked to her for at least forty-five minutes without stop. And here's the miraculous part: she attended to my every word, and even reached out her small hand to touch me at one point. She tracked the sound of my voice with her deep focus on my lips. She engaged fully in our dialogue, just nonverbally. I had no idea how such a small being, with such limited life experience, could possibly absorb all of the energy I was sending in her direction. Not only did she receive it, but she was able to give it back. As they say, "She had me at hello."

Later that day, Sonia grew cranky and started to cry. The nurses and my sister speculated that our time together had over-stimulated her. I fell into despair, but I pulled myself out of it quickly so that my sister and her husband would not have to take care of me on top of everything else. I very much wanted to be useful, so I left the hospital and got takeout dinner for everyone from a nearby diner—not asking if I should, not asking what folks wanted, just doing it without fanfare. It was a small token, but something accessible, universal, and ultimately needed. Much later that evening, when my sister and her husband went home and actually ate, I knew they were not tasting the food. They were numb and emotionally drained, yet they sat and nourished themselves, knowing they needed to find a way to get up the next day and return to the hospital, now the parents of one daughter who was alive and one son who had passed away in his father's arms hours before.

A few days later I returned to California, leaving my sister, brother-in-law, and baby niece. Physically, I was on the other side of the country. Emotionally and spiritually, I was in the NICU. I had been on a journey that altered my life forever and had no way to share it with those at home. I walked, I talked, but my heart was not the same. Looking at me from the outside, no one could know that I was shattered. For the first time in my life, I understood people who choose to live close to their parents and siblings.

/

As she grew, it was clear to all who met her that Sonia was not the type of baby to smile and coo. She was tough on folks; tough on me. After she came home from the hospital, when I would visit, I'd smile and try to engage her with toys and peek-a-boo and key rings and books, but she wasn't interested. Mainly she was interested in either Mom or Dad, which isn't that unusual. But having been around a lot of toddlers, I always prided myself on being able to get a laugh or a smile. Sonia did not indulge me. It was as if she'd already had a hard-enough life, enduring so much, that she was over playing the baby role and accommodating what adults wanted of her—a "been there, done that" kind of attitude.

But after that intimate moment in the NICU, I knew she and I were destined to be close. Living six hours away by plane did not make things easy, but every six months either my sister or I would make the cross-country trip.

For Sonia's first birthday, my sister and her husband traveled to Turks and Caicos with Sonia for a twofold purpose: to celebrate Sonia's first birthday and to spread the ashes of her twin brother. I met them there in the Caribbean, knowing the trip would be heart-wrenching. It was. The evening of my arrival, before I headed to my hotel room, my sister gave me a small bundle—a vivid blue cloth holding a coin-sized amount of Kai's ashes. I slept with the bundle placed against my heart. The humid air surrounded me as I lay thinking about all the joy we would never get to share. I kept the sliding door open so I could hear the ocean. It lulled me to sleep, a fitful slumber of jetlag and despair.

The next morning as I walked to the site where we were to spread Kai's ashes, I sobbed. It was the first time I had let myself feel the truth of what was about to happen. When I got to the spot where the others waited, I realized I could not separate from the only part of him I had. I asked my sister's permission *not* to spread the ashes and instead bring them back with me to the Pacific Ocean for my husband and two sons to take part in some farewell ritual. She understood. Truth be told, it's now been five years and I still have his ashes. Yes, I did spread a small amount in the Pacific, but I've kept the rest. I simply can't let go.

On the same day that the others spread Kai's ashes into the aquamarine water of Turks and Caicos, I watched Sonia stick her entire one-year-old face in a small chocolate cake and my heart filled with joy. I still wonder how a heart can hold so much sorrow and so much jubilation at the same time.

/

Sonia has a stuffed animal named Lovey. Once when I was visiting her, she explained that there were actually two Loveys: "the old Lovey" and "the new Lovey." The latter spoke French, rode a motorcycle, had tattoos, and donned a black leather jacket. As she outlined his exploits, it became clear that this new Lovey went on wild adventures and appeared to live a bohemian lifestyle. How a three-and-a-half-year-old created an alter ego for her more traditional, old-school comrade-in-arms escapes me, yet this is one of the things I love about my niece—her boundless imagination.

Her creativity doesn't end with playtime. It turns out, one of Sonia's favorite activities is having books read to her, and one of my favorite activities is reading to children. On our visits, we'd sit and I'd read. Before she could talk, I'd say, "Turn the page now," and she'd dutifully swipe the page on cue. Once she could speak, she'd recite the words on each page, having memorized every sentence of her favorite books even though she couldn't read yet.

In 2018, my writer friend Alexandria Giardino published the children's book *Ode to an Onion: Pablo Neruda and His Muse*, and I dutifully sent Sonia a copy. I'd made her a promise in the NICU that someday we would read Neruda together, and somewhere deep inside I knew she was waiting for me to make good on it. And I was right. My sister tells me that for a two-week stretch, that was the only book Sonia wanted to read.

When I can't visit in person, I stay in touch from a distance. But Sonia doesn't like video calling very much. She's someone who makes assessments about people through real-life reflective observation: no cameras, no screens. In person, she quickly picks up on nonverbal clues and will scold her mom if she catches her spacing out during their make-believe play time. Technology does not allow for that level of intimacy, so it's of little use to Sonia. While I admire her skill at sizing people up and her disdain for anything trying to imitate an in-person relationship, it makes it hard to stay connected.

When the COVID-19 pandemic began, my thoughts raced to New York. Sonia can't go out to play and preschool is closed; her whole life has been unsettled. It was hard enough for my sister and her husband to help Sonia adapt to the preschool routine. She'd enter the room and observe everything, preferring to stay on the sidelines and take it all in. Just as she was finally embracing active socialization and the school routine, sheltering in place took over her life. She's supposed to be getting ready for kindergarten in the fall. Now I wonder what she'll be doing.

In April 2020, I was supposed to meet up with my sister and Sonia on the East Coast to depart for our nephew's wedding aboard a cruise ship. Not anymore! Getting on a plane to visit in the near future seems out of the question; I cannot imagine exposing her to any unnecessary risk. Life feels even more complicated now when it comes to long-distance relationships of all sorts. As Sonia moves toward her fifth birthday, much of the United States is still sheltering in place. I have no definite date for seeing her in person. It's hard to be a good auntie when you can't be with your niece. But that doesn't mean I won't try my best.

Realizing it would be a while before I saw Sonia again in person and wanting to find a way to stay connected, I began videotaping myself reading stories to her. In the first one, I donned a parrot hat at the moment the character in the story mentioned her pet parrot. Each day, I'd find a creative way to make the story come alive across the miles. Another time, I read a story I had written myself, instead of a published book. Despite her misgivings about video calls, Sonia enjoys watching my videos. I was thrilled to find out that she asked to see one of the stories I read *twice*. Eventually, I realized I could make the stories available to my other nieces and, ultimately, I began a YouTube channel, Storytelling with Tia Maria, so that any children sheltering in place could watch them.

Sonia had become my muse. And along the way, this little person, born weighing a mere two pounds, has grown into a true heavyweight. I'm ever so grateful to have her in my life and in my corner.

What I Carry

BY TYRESE COLEMAN

The last time I entered a neonatal intensive care unit I had a panic attack. One of my friends had just birthed thirty-weeker twins who were incubated at a hospital outside of Philadelphia. Another Catholic hospital, I thought, as I entered the futuristically gothic space of modern glass doors, dark wood arches, and crucifixes.

It's hard now to recall the true image of that NICU; it seemed tacked-on to the side or rear of the hospital. My mind conjures an atmosphere more foreboding than reality; my emotions taint the image in my head. When I close my eyes, I see a place more like an old sanatorium: yellowed-white walls, hallways leading to darkened rooms containing not just beeping monitors or whooshing oxygen tanks but ghosts and phantoms cloudy with illness. I see an asylum offering no refuge.

My friends and I sat in the waiting room until the new father came out to meet us. When we were buzzed in, a cold wave floated up and spread over my body. The memory of that click, the sound that signaled you'd reached the gateway to your children, triggered an awful familiarity. It wasn't a comforting awareness, like the smell of your child's hair or the feel of his bare feet laid against your cheek. It was a tiny alarm, warning you of the dangers ahead.

Still, I followed the others; we entered, rounding the corner. There: The nurses' station. The sink. The hospital-grade foam soap. All the same as our NICU, four years before. My entire body tensed when I turned on the water and began performing that innocuous task of washing my hands. It's a task I do every single day of my life. A task I did over and over again each time

I wanted to see my children, for more than three and a half months. The same smell. The same airy density of the foam. The feel of it coating my hands, and the half-warm water dissolving it away.

It became hard for me to breathe. Hard for me to hold back the tears throbbing for release. I sobbed, fanning my face rapidly with my wet hand, stammering words to my friends that I cannot recall. Instantly embarrassed, yet unable to control myself, all I wanted was escape. I had to get out of there.

/

Having a baby is traumatic, even in a normal pregnancy. A foreign body grows inside your own. The pain and ripping-apart of your insides as you bring forth this being into the world, ultimately destroying the life you had prior to that moment. In an instant, you, the person you have been all of your life, dies. I don't mean this to sound morose, but I wish to acknowledge the gravity of childbirth. I wish to show how, at any moment, you can slip away—right in the midst of the pushing, or while spread on a surgical table, your lower body paralyzed. Slip away from who you are, who you were. Slip away from life itself. Since the beginning of time, childbirth has been a dangerous undertaking. It has killed people much stronger than me.

I don't know which trauma spurred my self-diagnosed PTSD: birthing babies at twenty-five weeks or watching my children fight for their lives for more than three and a half months. But I know it is rooted in the NICU. And I know I'm not the only one. Approximately 10 to 15 percent of people who give birth—even under normal circumstances—develop postpartum depression (PPD). However, those who give birth to premature babies have a significantly higher risk of developing PPD. Studies have shown that as many as 40 percent of women who give birth to premature babies suffer from PPD, and many partners also develop depression and post-traumatic stress.

I am one of them.

Having preemies, for me, was a waiting game, and I have never been good at waiting. Waiting on hospital bed rest to give birth to my babies, knowing they would be born far too early, waiting to find out what would happen to them. And then another, even more helpless waiting: walking into the NICU every day, wondering how much longer they would be there, how much more I could take. It's a trauma that rolls on and on.

My children came into the world under fearful circumstances and lived the earliest part of their lives in a state of uncertainty. For NICU parents—constantly exposed to the sounds of emergency, the iron smell of blood, the cries of babies you are unable to console even when they are your own—such impotence is life. There are babies coding, doctors telling other anxious, suffering parents terrible news in hushed tones. There is sobbing— sometimes muffled, sometimes rending. You long to hold your children, to take them and run as far away as you can, but you know their best hope lies in the sterile isolettes, the endlessly beeping machines, the practiced efficiency of doctors and nurses. And so you stay, and you absorb the fear and uncertainty all around you. What other choice do you have?

After three and half months we left the NICU. But the NICU never left us.

/

I had been back to my sons' NICU only once since they were released: a holiday party when they were about two years old. The hospital's social worker emailed us about these events occasionally. They were meant to bring current NICU families and NICU graduate families together, to give those still living through this trauma a glimpse of a different reality—and, for graduates, a form of peer support and a way to cope with PTSD.

It didn't work for me. Walking back through the doors meant walking right back into the feelings that had lurked beneath the surface for two years.

Across the room, I saw the spiky gray hair of one of our NICU doctors bobbing up and down near the front door. Just seeing her face instantly brought tears down my own. She was the doctor who told me I needed to prepare myself for the death of one of my babies, while I was on hospital bed rest. She asked me then: did I want to risk both of their lives by having them early or did I want to save one and let the other die? A choice that was no choice at all. And, later, she was the doctor who told me necrotizing enterocolitis was the leading cause of death for preemies—when she diagnosed my baby boy with it.

I remember being grateful for her bluntness, for the fact that she respected me enough to tell me the hard truth, no sugar-coating. That, I imagine, is how a NICU doctor has to live her life to get through so much trauma every day. One cannot sugarcoat death.

But now, seeing her face erased the past two years, and I was right back there, waiting by my sons' bedsides, wondering what traumatic news she would bring us next. We stayed at the party for less than thirty minutes.

I haven't gone back to that hospital since.

/

There are tangible reminders we hold on to as preemie parents.

I've kept some trinkets from their plastic-box days. There are the two tiny gift-shop stuffed animals I used to measure their growth. One is a blue bear with his hands together in prayer. I would put the bear next to my boys, see how over the weeks it went from being larger than my babies to half their size by the time they were released. I can fit the bear inside the palm of my hand.

I have the blankets their grandmother quilted, short squares just the right size to cover their isolettes and block out the harsh hospital lighting. I have their hospital ID ankle bracelets; leftover circular bandages to hold their oxygen tubes in place on their cheeks; tiny knit hats that had been donated to the hospital to help regulate their temperatures.

I saved them, these reminders I can touch to bring back each and every day we spent inside the NICU, the items of their infancy I keep with love, regardless of the suffering that taints them.

But there are intangible reminders, too.

In his short story about the trauma of the Vietnam War, "The Things They Carried," Tim O'Brien writes, "To carry something was to hump it . . . In its intransitive form, to hump meant to walk, or to march, but it implied burdens far beyond the intransitive."

His use of the word "intransitive" is curious. Intransitive verbs do not contain a direct object, but the verb "to carry" is transitive and requires an object to make sense in a sentence. Grammatically, one carries something; one does not simply *carry*.

But I do. I carry these intangibles. I imagine my PTSD inside a sack thrown across a shoulder, a load so heavy my body bends at the waist from the weight of it. What we lug around inside our bodies and then inside our minds, our memories. What we clench to us with everything but our hands.

I've kept the fear, the nightmares, the anger, and the guilt close to my heart every day since my sons' birth. I developed a fear of going near water, afraid the boys might fall or be pushed into it and taken from me forever.

And that is the basis of it, lodged so deep within me I think I will carry it until the day I die. The fear of losing them. It has the smell of antiseptic foam soap, the sound of automatic hospital doors opening, the feel of lukewarm water splashing over my hands. I've humped these intangibles, these intransitives, with me since the day they were born.

/

If you had told me that instead of walking into my friend's hospital and going straight back to see her babies, I'd explode, feel my heart beat out of my chest, hyperventilate, and weep, I would have said you were mistaken. But it was I who was mistaken. Because when I think on it, this scene was inevitable, this dropping of composure and resolve I'd propped myself up against for years. I'd cultivated a sense of normalcy, just another thing that I carried.

It had been almost four years since I'd seen the inside of a NICU. Four years since I spent days crouched between my boys' twin plastic boxes, since I'd placed my pinky inside their minuscule palms and watched as their fingers did not even wrap all the way around when curled. Four years removed from the constant noise, the anxiety from alarms, from fearing for their lives before they even truly began.

Time is a manipulator, making me think that the longer I am away from a place that caused so much fear and guilt and pain means that I would eventually be over that fear, that guilt, and that pain. Or rather, maybe I tried to manipulate time, made it an escape, an out, for not addressing the trauma of the NICU like I should have. I let the years and the fears accumulate until the day I was confronted with them once more, when I began reckoning with everything I had carried for so long.

/

But time does more than trick us. It also turned my tiny sons into little boys long past preemie-hood. Early on the sunny January day that I visited my friend, I went through the routine that had become remarkably un-noteworthy: I packed their lunches, saw one son onto his school bus, and then did the same for his brother.

Time no longer ticks by in pulse-oximeter stats, or the minutes between bradycardias, or the steady beep beep beep of a heart-rate monitor. Now it moves as thirty-minute episodes of Doc McStuffins and eating Cheerios at the kitchen counter. It passes as seasons, first days of school, birthday parties.

Time carries us.

Destination: Okay

BY JANINE KOVAC

On the day of my twins' two-month vaccinations, I received emails from two different websites.

According to the pregnancy website, my babies were still fetuses. "At thirty-three weeks pregnant," the email read, "you are probably thinking about your baby's delivery. If you haven't already, you need to start preparing to go to the hospital at any moment. Even though your due date is seven weeks away, you want to be prepared for any pregnancy complications that may occur, such as premature labor."

The other email, from a parenting website, informed me of the "normal milestones" two-month-olds reach. "Babies at this age like to look at colors and patterns," it read.

My three-year-old daughter had been that kind of baby—reaching for toys dangled in front of her. But my two-month-old twin boys were in the neonatal intensive care unit, where they would stay for another month. Michael and Wagner were born at twenty-five weeks and four days on December 30, 2009. Michael weighed one pound, twelve ounces. His brother weighed just over a pound and a half. They both had surgeries, on the same day, to correct two patent ductus arteriosus (PDAs) in their hearts at three weeks of age. Only a few brain bleeds, not too serious. Bradycardias and apneas? Far too many to count. At two months old they were still on oxygen, still fed through a nasogastric tube.

My husband and I knew they were doing well by micropreemie standards, but we also knew that we had to hold two sets of ages in our heads: chronological and adjusted. Chronological age was used on official documents, such as birth certificates and insurance claims. Adjusted age accounted for their prematurity in order to have a more accurate marker for their development. Until their mid-April due date, the boys would be counted in gestational weeks. After that, they'd be tracked as if they were newborns. When it came to developmental milestones, we were told, we would probably need to subtract three to four months from their chronological age for the next two or three years.

We were on two roads at the same time. The first was the road to health. Our twins were on a medical journey where ventilators and heart monitors compensated for their underdeveloped organs. Trained professionals stood at the helm of complicated medical equipment. They adjusted dials for oxygen and recorded data. My husband and I sat by our boys' bedsides and worried about possible futures. Would they have physical disabilities, cognitive ones, or both? When would we know? Was there something that could be done to change a difficult future into an optimal one? What did "optimal" even mean when you are born three and a half months early?

Then there was the parent journey. We held our babies as often as possible. We cooed in baby talk so they'd know our voices. We dressed them in preemie clothes and took pictures for their baby album. These moments weren't about the future. They were about holding our babies heart-to-heart and feeling their warmth. We loved our boys because they were ours, and in those moments, that's all that mattered.

I couldn't shake the sensation that I always had to look at my boys from two vantage points—where they were and where they ought to be. But I was afraid that if I just charted their progress (or lack thereof), then I'd miss the best moments of being a mom. I started a diary to keep track of it all.

/

March 27, 2010

We are truly in the home stretch. We moved to Nursery 3 (where the big five-pounders are). Both boys have been off oxygen for over a week and are getting all their feeds by breast or bottle.

I am also getting quizzed by the nurses at every turn. Just walking to the fridge to get fresh milk I have to field three or four trivia questions:

When your baby sits up at seven months, how old is he really? (Four months.)

How old, in both corrected and biological months, do you expect your baby to be when he walks? (One year; fifteen months.)

In August, how old will your baby really be? (Five months.)

In fact, even though they are almost three months old now, we are still counting in gestational weeks. (They will be thirty-eight weeks this Sunday.) It's easy to look at them now and think of them as newborn babies and not as three-month-olds, but months from now, it will be hard not to compare their progress with other December babies. The nurses hurl their corrected-age questions because they want us to remember that the twins are actually April babies.

It feels like the week before school lets out. And then the fun really begins, right?

Oh! Wagner just hit six pounds and Michael's not far behind at five pounds & thirteen ounces. They're almost four times their original birth weight!

/

Our NICU doctors and nurses conspicuously avoided the word "normal." Instead they used phrases such as "typically developing" or "significant differences." I was grateful for their semantic choices. No part of this experience, from pregnancy to our three-month NICU stay, had felt "normal." This was not my picture of motherhood.

Then again, the word "normal" had always bristled me. Even

before I had micropreemie twins, I equated "normal" with "average" and "ordinary." By that definition, I never wanted to be normal. I wanted to stand out. I spent a dozen years as a professional ballet dancer elbowing my way to claim center stage. Later, when I went to college, I fought to graduate at the top of my class, even though I was almost twenty years older than my classmates. I wanted to be special and that meant clawing to the top.

I wanted my children to be special, too. I had high hopes that my daughter Chiara (a healthy term baby born weighing seven pounds) would be the fastest crawler, the strongest walker, the smartest toddler. The baby books told me it was not a race. But to me it was, and I wanted us to finish first.

It was hard work to read the latest research on baby sign language and find the best infant massage techniques, but I was motivated by the payoff of a baby genius. At Mom-and-Baby yoga class, I kept a careful eye on the other infants. I knew which seven-monthers had already pulled themselves up to standing and which eight-month-olds should have been crawling already but weren't.

I kept an eye on the other mothers, too. Were they as tired as I was? The unstructured days of early motherhood spent tending to the needs of my baby made me restless and exhausted at the same time. My swollen postpartum body bore little resemblance to the sinewy figure I'd had as a ballet dancer. I hoped that a few downward dogs might bring me back to my old self. The moms around me had gray faces and slouched shoulders, just like me. Would they get back in shape before I did? Everything was a contest.

Despite the stroller I bought to strengthen my baby's budding core muscles and the special brain exercises we practiced to a soundtrack of Mozart, Chiara hit all of her milestones within the "normal" range. It was clear that she was not going to be a child prodigy. I stopped acting like Baby's Personal Trainer. I was irked that she was perfectly normal and therefore perfectly ordinary, but honestly, I just wasn't willing to put in the work if my efforts weren't having any noticeable effect. I erased "Destination: Brilliant" from my map of motherhood milestones.

/

Wednesday, July 14, 2010

The boys are now three months old adjusted. They are HUGE. Weighing in at thirteen pounds, six ounces, Michael is seven times his birth weight. Wagner weighs thirteen pounds, or eight times his birth weight. They are both twenty-four inches long, or twice as long as they were the day they were born (six and a half months ago). They are doing great. And we're still doing a lot of work to make sure it stays that way.

Our big thing to work on now is grabbing toys, but the twins don't really care about that. They are far more interested in faces, particularly Mama's, Daddy's, and Chiara's. They are transfixed by Chiara's face.

But the best was the other day—both boys were lying on our bed. It was right before the late afternoon nap and they hadn't quite settled in yet, so they were making those noncommittal cries that make you think, "Should I pick them up or what?"

Chiara climbed onto the bed and sat between them. She put a hand on the chest of each baby.

"It's okay. You're okay," she said in a soothing voice. "I'm right here."

/

When the twins were ten months old (six and a half months adjusted), I decided to load up all three kids and head to Mom-and-Baby yoga. I wasn't sure how much of the class I'd be able to take, but that wasn't the point. The point was to show off my preschooler and her brothers. We had come so far in such a short time. Both boys were sitting up unassisted. They could support their weight on all fours, rocking back and forth and showing signs of crawling. They were even starting to show an interest in real food.

The teacher introduced us to the class. "Here's a Mom-and-Baby alumna!" she said of Chiara, who grinned sheepishly and hid behind my legs.

"And look at these guys! I can't believe they were born three months early and weighing less than two pounds!"

There were audible gasps. One mother actually shielded her baby as if extreme prematurity were contagious.

"Living miracles." The teacher shook her head. "Well, welcome back. They look great."

She didn't ask how old the twins were, and I was grateful. I never knew what to say. It felt misleading to give their adjusted age and they were obviously too small and too stationary for their chronological age.

I arranged my yoga mat and gave my daughter a bag of carrot sticks to munch on. I was the only person with more than one baby, and judging from the gawks of the others, the only mother of preemies. I could feel their pity aimed at me from behind a wall of insincere smiles. I could feel their silent sighs of relief, too. I was sure they were all thinking how grateful they were not to be in my shoes (or, in this case, bare feet).

I felt a pang of resentment and then a twinge of shame. It wasn't that long ago—and in this very room—that I'd been that condescending mother, thinly disguising my relief behind a sympathetic nod.

As hard as it was to ignore the mothers, it was even harder to ignore the other babies. Each one shone like a little spotlight. Some were just newborns, saffron bundles sleeping soundly in their car seats, while others sat like potted plants. Still others were rolling or crawling, signaling their imminent graduation from the Mom-and-Baby class.

The ones in car seats who were more blanket than baby were

likely around six weeks old. The ones grabbing at toys that dangled from their play mats would be between two and four months old. Rolling over was the next gross motor stage, which in most babies, occurred around four months. Next came sitting unassisted, which was not impressive to look at, but I knew was essential for building the core strength necessary to crawl, stand, and walk.

Knowing that I wasn't supposed to compare my babies didn't make it any easier.

All of those other babies looked so ... normal. It wasn't just the gross motor skills they exhibited. I could see how the potted plants and the ones grabbing at toys were also hitting the typical developmental milestones for cognitive abilities. The younger ones snapped to attention when they heard their mothers' voices. My twins should have been doing that months ago. The older ones could follow their mothers' gazes, and in some cases, even babble responses. My twins should have been doing that, too.

Suddenly I wished I hadn't come. This was supposed to be a victory lap. But looking at my boys, I felt hopelessly far behind.

/

February 25, 2011

It's official. The boys have language delays. They are nearly fourteen months old (ten and a half months adjusted) and they still don't know any words. By ten months, Chiara had already said her first word and was starting to use sign language regularly.

I don't mean that the boys don't say any words; I mean that the boys don't understand any words. They don't turn to me when someone says, "Where's Mama?" They don't know who "Daddy" is. When you say, "Look!" and point, they don't look. They don't even know their own names, a milestone that is usually reached around six months of age.

We are way off that mark.

/

March 2, 2011

I'm starting to get concerned. I haven't yet been able to talk to the speech therapist from our NICU Early Intervention playgroup because the boys have not been healthy enough to attend since November. They haven't been that sick (except for this week—this week three out of four ears are infected and we have just been given a fancy three-day second-line antibiotic. Last night Mister Wagner ran a 104.5 temperature). It's just that the playgroup is all NICU grads—in other words, babies with fragile immune systems. Even thinking of attending when all three of us are less than 100 percent healthy isn't just bad form, it's dangerous for the other babies.

I talked to the speech therapist associated with our new developmental playgroup (the one run by Chiara's daycare). She's very nice and very respected, but she had never met our babies before two Fridays ago. Her suggestion was to "bombard them with language" and she previewed for me a storm of sounds and "power signs" to help jumpstart our wordless tots.

/

Even the experts don't fully understand how we acquire language. They just know that it happens. If you're around it, it will come. There are about two hundred different consonant and vowel sounds across all of the languages spoken in the world. When babies are born, they are attuned to each of these phonological sounds. But as they learn their soon-to-be-native language, they come to hear only that language's subset of sounds and to block out the others.

As babies start to tease out the noise around them, they also start to figure out that strings of speech sounds correlate to certain meanings. Around the six-month mark, most babies figure out that there is a string of sounds that correlates to *them*. Around that age, when typically developing babies hear their name, they turn their heads to look at the speaker.

They learn from context, too. "All gone" is consistently said at the end of a meal. "Uh-oh" after something is dropped. "Bye-bye," "Night-night," and "Look!" are also regularly repeated in the same contexts. Babies on the verge of learning words are also good at determining intentionality. That means they can tell the difference between when Dad looks at Baby and says, "There's your bottle!" and when Dad looks at Baby but is really saying to Mom, "There's your cell phone!"

Nearly a month had passed since I first noticed what the boys weren't noticing—their names, our names, simple commands such as "Come here," "Look!," and "No!" They were approaching fifteen months old—not quite a year adjusted. It was hard not to remember how precocious Chiara had been when she was learning to talk. By her first birthday, she had several baby signs: "more," "please," "thank you," and even "help." She had a handful of words and she seemed to understand everything. My husband and I learned the hard way that words such as "cookie," "ice cream," or "go to the park" to our daughter's ear were as precious as promises and were words better left unsaid unless we were prepared to follow through.

Michael and Wagner showed none of this understanding. Well-meaning friends and neighbors shared anecdotes about someone in their family (always an uncle, strangely enough) who never said a word until he was three or four or even five years old, at which point he spoke in complete sentences. But surely Uncle X communicated in other ways. Was that acquired later, too?

Around this time, we noticed something else: Because of their exposure to incessant noise during their NICU stay, the twins didn't startle. Sudden noises did not surprise or scare them. If I clapped my hands or dropped a book out of their line of sight, the twins would not turn in the direction of the noise.

We knew they could hear. As with Chiara, our boys had trained us to tiptoe after we put them down to sleep. And there were other noises that grabbed their attention, such as the mechanical notes on a favorite toy or the rumbling of the garbage truck outside. Hearing tests with a pediatric audiologist confirmed they could hear. The issue, then, was that while the ears sent signals to the brain, the signals did not elicit a response.

Now instead of two roads, the medical and parent journeys, I felt like a third developmental journey had been added.

The road to health seemed simple. There were regular check-ups to schedule and attend. There were timetables to follow and symptoms to look out for. Vaccines for respiratory syncytial virus (RSV), antibiotics for ear infections, diaper cream for rashes. There was an answer for everything. The parent road was simple, too. There were no timetables or expectations. The only thing required of me was that I show up and love them as they were. I cuddled my babies. We had tickle games in our big bed and excursions to the park.

But the language delays introduced a new wrinkle. What if it wasn't enough to bombard them with words? What if they weren't like all those uncles who suddenly started monologizing at age four? What if this was just the way my babies were?

For the first year of the boys' post-NICU life, we attended a weekly playgroup facilitated by early intervention specialists. The sessions rotated over four topics: gross motor skills, fine motor skills, speech, and general development. Usually Wagner slept through them, but at least I could see how Michael was progressing with his pincher grip or his army crawl.

Here, caregivers (usually the mothers) came with their babies. Our only common thread was that we'd all been in the NICU, but each of us had a different back story. Here, babies progressed at their own rate—and, unlike my old Mom-and-Baby yoga class, I felt no judgment from (or toward) the other parents. I didn't even feel judgment toward my old type-A self. Back then, I measured steps and counted syllables. I was convinced that having a precocious toddler would make me look like a better mother. By contrast, in the NICU, I charted oxygen-saturation rates and counted heartbeats per minute, and it wasn't about me at all. The only goal was the ongoing process of how my boys could get the care they needed to thrive. I loved my kids. Disabilities and delays wouldn't change that; it would just change the support I gave them.

I was no longer gunning for "Destination: Brilliant." I wasn't trying to be a "better" mother. These days, when I reviewed the latest research on child development, it wasn't to teach my kids more; it was to figure out what they already knew.

Some days I wasn't sure which was the miracle: that my boys learned to breathe and survived extreme prematurity or that my daughter (and everyone else I knew) had mastered breathing without any machines to help. Knowing how hard my sons and other preemies worked to reach each milestone overwhelmed me with awe.

After a year of the early intervention group, the focus shifted to address the boys' language acquisition delays.

"Don't worry about the words," Cathy, the facilitator, told us, contradicting the advice of a previous speech therapist. "First, we're going to learn to take turns."

Cathy sat next to Wagner, looking him in the eye. He was more interested in digging Cheerios crumbs out of the carpet. She continued to stare. Finally, Wagner looked up. Cathy smiled and patted her leg twice. She watched her own gesture and then she looked at Wagner. Then she did it again. And again. And again.

Each time, Wagner watched her. He looked at her hand. He looked at her face. After several minutes, Cathy said, "That's enough for today. We'll do it again next week."

Before you use words, you must understand that someone wishes to talk to you. You must understand when it is your turn to speak. You must understand what is expected of you—are you expected to get the ball? Are you expected to answer the question? Are you expected to keep listening? Imagine a waiter who makes eye contact and nods, but never comes over to your table. He has communicated something to you that makes you expect something from him, but he has done something entirely different.

The following month at the playgroup, I pushed the twins' stroller through the labyrinth of halls. In the distance, a tiny baby wailed the hungry cry of a newborn. Michael jerked his head in the direction of the noise and scanned the room until he saw its source—a bundle in a stroller at the far end of the room.

I unfastened their belts and lifted each twin out of the stroller and onto the floor. Michael crawled toward the baby. His interest waned when the babe's mother unbuttoned her shirt to feed her child. Wagner crawled over to Cathy, who sat on the carpet near the toddler toys. He patted her leg twice and smiled.

Cathy caught my eye. She didn't say anything, but her grin told me everything I needed to know.

/

May 23, 2011

Today, Michael went over to the bench where we keep jackets and shoes, rummaged through the jackets, and tossed his brother's shoes to the floor until he found what he was looking for: his own shoes. He brought them over to me and turned around and sat in my lap, his way of asking me to put his shoes on so he could go outside.

At almost seventeen months (thirteen-and-a-half adjusted), it is his most complete act of communication to date.

I just sat there and cried.

/

November 10, 2011

We watch the twins carefully to make sure they're not too delayed.

Everything seems to be going well. They have some language delays, but they are progressing—just enough to make us feel like we should stop worrying but not enough to actually keep us from worrying.

We have been holding our breaths for the next milestone: two-word sentences. (They are twenty-two months old now.)

Today, Wagner said his second two-word sentence (his first two-word sentence was "my turn"). We were at the toddler park and he went down the little toddler slide, which he has done by himself about a million times, but this time he did a little tumble at the bottom.

When he got up and dusted himself off, he told himself, "You're okay."

/

In truth, I wasn't sure if "You're okay" meant Wagner was comforting himself or if he was simply repeating a string of sounds he'd heard us say to him. But I counted the milestones anyway. For language: a novel instance of a two-word sentence. For social-emotional development: self-consolation. Gross motor skills: balance and coordination. Well, sort of.

I sat on the wood chips and watched as Wagner wobbled back to the slide, undeterred by his stumble. I'd never seen him do that before, but something about it was so familiar—so *Wagner*.

A memory tugged at the edge of my mind. Wagner, at just a week old. His weight had dropped to hover at the one-pound mark. He'd had a pulmonary hemorrhage—blood in his lungs. Doctors couldn't tell us why it had happened or if it would happen again. When I got the call, I rushed to the hospital. I felt helpless and hopeless. I was sure that he was going to die.

The nurse showed me how to saturate a long cotton swab with breast milk. Wagner was too fragile to be picked up. In fact,

I wouldn't be able to hold him for another two weeks. But when I extended the swab through the doors of his isolette, he turned toward me, eyes still closed. He smacked his lips and opened his mouth. Even when he was at his weakest, he was still ready to take on the world.

Now, as I watched him dust himself off and try again, I could see how that personality was present even as a week-old one-pounder. And Michael, too. The toddler who'd brought me his shoes, demanding to go outside, was very much the same micropreemie who'd tugged on his tubes and fidgeted during diaper changes. Even when they were at their most vulnerable, they were still *them*. All the work we had done, everything we were doing to strengthen their motor skills and communication and social skills, only helped them express what was inside them all along.

At some point, the twins' road to health converged with my motherhood journey. Yeah, it was taking us a while to speak and learn and listen. But I was okay with that. These boys—my boys—were always there right in front me and I was always there for them. When it came to love, we were right on target.

I'm trying not to conclude with a cheesy, "Yes, it's all going to be okay." But quite frankly, I can't think of anything better.

Past the Limits

BY MANUEL HERNANDEZ

I was born in Colombia, on the northwestern coast of South America, facing the Caribbean. My mother was in her twenty-fifth week of pregnancy when she developed pre-eclampsia, a life-threatening medical condition characterized by really high blood pressure during pregnancy. She was at work as a receptionist at the time, but her coworkers told her she must go to the hospital immediately. I was born that night. I was the smallest baby she and my father had ever held.

I stopped breathing three times in my first few hours because my lungs were extremely underdeveloped. I was connected to a ventilator and put under critical care. The doctors gave me seventy-two hours to live. A nurse told my mother that if I were to survive this, I would suffer complications and could be left in an unresponsive state. Perhaps she believed she was doing a panicked mother a favor by being pragmatic, but in my mother's opinion, that nurse lacked the tact and compassion she needed at the time. Miraculously, after twenty-five days in the neonatal intensive care unit, I survived. The worst persistent health condition I have is my asthma, probably due to my underdeveloped lungs.

When I was seven years old, in the second grade, my mother and I emigrated to join my father, who was working here in the United States. Over time, I began to realize my parents had emigrated for my sake, so that I could have all of the benefits this country has to offer. At the time, the main benefit was education. The more educated you are, the more options and advantages you have in life, my parents would say.

When we first moved here, I knew zero English, but I picked it up fairly quickly. In school, they put me in English for Speakers of Other Languages, or ESOL, classes. Before I knew it—after only half a year of living in the United States—I was thinking in both English and Spanish. Maybe I learned the language quickly because of my age and neuroplasticity; I knew some ESOL students in high school who had a harder time learning the language. It also helped that the majority of students in my elementary school were Hispanic. It was a melting pot of races and cultures in one academic system. Making friends was easy; other bilingual students helped me out a lot and made me feel welcome.

I arrived in the United States on a visa and overstayed its expiration to participate in my primary education. When I was seventeen, I went through the complex and expensive process of becoming a naturalized citizen. My uncle, an American citizen, had helped support my family since we arrived in the country. The four of us, including my parents, had become our own family. My uncle and my parents decided that the best way for me to stay in this country would be for him to adopt me so I could become a citizen. There was already a history of love and trust between us all. It seemed only natural for him to adopt me to give me the opportunities that my parents wouldn't be able to provide—everything made possible by citizenship: higher education, job opportunities, insurance, a better life. That word, *opportunities*, came up a lot throughout the process. I would not be where I am today if not for the kindness of my uncle.

I don't know if it was hard for my parents to let my uncle adopt me; it never seemed appropriate to ask, but I imagine it was a hard decision to make. I could ask, but to be honest, I have no desire to know. I understand why they did it, and I'm sure they don't regret it, especially when I received my bachelor's degree.

To become a naturalized citizen, I was given a study booklet on basic American history and how our democracy works. It felt like a review from middle school. The staff at the citizenship resource center was very helpful. I answered questions, including about any ties to terrorist organizations—don't worry, I never had any. On a freezing, snowy day, I dressed up very formally in a suit and tie to receive the certificate documenting my status as an American citizen. My family proudly attended the ceremony. There was a prerecorded video of President Trump congratulating the new American citizens, the irony of which created a noticeably awkward mood in the auditorium, with some staff and even white families rolling their eyes.

My parents are still undocumented, and it worries me—especially when I hear stories of other undocumented immigrant families and the racists who call U.S. Immigration and Customs Enforcement (ICE) on them. At any time, my parents could be pulled away from me and sent back to a country they have not lived in for decades.

/

When it was time to leave high school, I had no idea what I wanted to do with my life. It seemed as though from childhood to my teenage years, almost everything had been decided for me. Not necessarily in a bad way, because my parents and teachers and counselors did their best to guide me, and everyone wanted the best for me. But the fact that I had little experience making my own choices also meant it was harder to know what I wanted to do. I imagine many people go through similar feelings of apprehension and uncertainty after graduation.

I thought of picking up a job in the trades, maybe as an electrician or a plumber, because I didn't want to go through the college process. Everybody tried to talk me out of that—my parents, their friends, my school counselors. Looking back, seeing all of the employment benefits electricians have, I really think it might have been a good career choice. But I don't regret being pushed to go to community college and eventually university, because it led to the path I'm on now, in media and film.

At times, I've felt pressure—as an only child, as the child of immigrants, as a miracle baby, as the son my parents would do anything for. The pressure comes from wanting to succeed, to live up to expectations, to go above and beyond for my family. I suppose every child faces certain expectations. But when you know your parents have worked extremely hard for your education, you feel the responsibility to make something of yourself so that you can eventually give back to them in some way. There was also the pressure as a first-generation student to prove myself.

But I was really apprehensive about what I might get myself into by going to college. I didn't want to go into debt when I didn't even know what my major might be. I was trying to find the truth for myself.

A friend of mine recommended going into business or accounting because, he said, the demand for those professions was high and a lot of money could be made. The logic made sense: study money, the exchange of it, and build a career in it. But when I started taking my first few business classes, I absolutely hated them—economics in particular. And, outside of my new academic life, I was working at my first two part-time jobs, in a department store and a local library, for more money in my pocket and to practice my newfound autonomy. But working so much meant I was falling behind in classes.

With very little direction and motivation, I fell into depression. I didn't even realize what depression was at the time; I thought it just meant feeling sad. I started skipping classes, oversleeping in the afternoons, reevaluating my life. I thought I was wasting my time in what felt like a second high school. My grades began to nose-dive, even in classes I loved, like psychology. It raised concerns with my psychology professor, who was also a licensed psychiatrist, to the point where he asked to meet with me during his office hours.

He was the first professor who seemed concerned about the way I was behaving (or was not behaving). When we met during his office hours, I told him why I was doing poorly. Every morning when I woke up, I felt paralyzed with no motivation to work or go to school. Maybe paralyzed is the wrong word, because it implies a stillness triggered by anxiety or fear. This was closer to feeling like a marionette with its strings cut, with no invisible hand to fix the strings or move the lifeless puppet. I didn't speak to my friends much. I was completely apathetic, and not even aware of it. I was finally an adult, finally living life on my own terms, but I found little joy and meaning in the things I did. "Is this what college and being an adult is supposed to feel like?" I asked. "I don't feel like this is how I should be spending my life, just doing something I don't want to do."

All of this just tumbled out. My professor told me it seemed like I was depressed. I was in my twenties, he said, and these years should be spent trying out new experiences and seeing what makes me happy. The mistake I made was truly believing that I could map out my life by going into accounting. Life should be more complex and fun than pursuing something you have no interest in. If everyone had what they wanted laid out from birth, there would be little room for surprise and growth. Talking to him helped me see that.

The professor asked me what I enjoyed doing—if there was anything in school that felt right to me. I told him I have always enjoyed creative writing. I was especially into television and film; when I was in high school, I would fantasize of being a novelist or a screenwriter. He recommended me for a creative writing class, and I eventually switched into the media and film program. For the first time in my life, I was excited to learn. Whether as a career or for recreation, I genuinely enjoy pursuing the arts.

Not everyone supported my decision. My friends would joke around about how I was going to be a starving artist, serving lattes at Starbucks for the rest of my life. I do know people who pursue the arts and support themselves by working at coffee shops, but it isn't horrifying like the jokes made it out to be. Those artists aren't "starving," either. I would rather do something meaningful to me than make a fortune as a stock trader. When I lacked support from my friends, my parents' encouragement was a safe haven. My parents are the only people who have always had my back. They saw how happy my new path made me, and they supported me all the way.

I always thought of the "American dream" as owning a home, but that isn't *my* American dream. I want to be a self-made man in my own right, free from debt, free to go to any state or country, no boundaries. For now, I want to pursue what I have been studying for so long. I want to create things I can be proud of.

I do feel pressure, though, to support my parents as they get older. They have provided the world for me. I want not only to surpass my family's expectations but to go beyond them. They deserve it. I am their only son, their miracle baby, and I hope someday to give them a life without pain or struggle or hard work. Often I wonder who I am living for: them or myself. Can it be both? I want to do so much with the life I have, the life they have helped me to make.

When I was younger, my parents would tell me about my origins—the circumstances of my birth and where I come from. I was too much of a rebellious kid then to appreciate what they said. I believed my existence should be determined by the present, not the past. But I understand, now, the miracle of my birth—and of my survival. It is scary to fathom I was at death's door before my very first words. To realize my whole timeline was at the mercy of God makes me appreciate what I have and not take anything for granted. It is still a little terrifying. I am where I am today not just because of my hard work but also because of everyone who made my life possible.

I still don't know exactly where this path will take me. My pragmatism and idealism constantly clash. The idealist points to the destination, and the pragmatist builds roadblocks along the way. I believe that everyone fears what they want the most, because if they pursue it, they might never get it. People impose limits on themselves. But in my life, I have already pushed past what seemed possible. I know I will face more and more challenges as I continue down this path. But I am fortunate to have a strong foundation, birthed from unforeseen circumstances.

Acknowledgments

First of all, I want to thank everyone who loves, supports, and helps preemie families: Our partners, friends, and families, and the teams of nurses, doctors, midwives, specialists, techs, doulas, and lactation consultants who have dedicated their lives to caring for our tiniest ones. We could not do this without our communities standing right behind us, lifting us up.

Editing this book has been a labor of love, and I'm so excited to see it arriving into the world. Endless thanks to Eric Smith and Ryan Harrington (and everyone at Melville House and Penguin Random) for understanding the importance of an anthology like this and striving to bring it to the widest possible audience.

Thank you to the contributors for spending your nights and weekends crafting and perfecting these essays. Thank you for believing in this book; thank you for sharing these stories; thank you for all the help and guidance and light you offer to other families. One of the greatest pleasures of creating this book has been getting to know all of you, which has made me a better writer and parent.

I also need to thank those who have been with me every step of the way, encouraging me back when this book idea was just a twinkle in my eye: Swapna Krishna, Ruthie Brown, Nicole Chung, Amanda Palleschi, Christine Grimaldi (Nonfiction Row!), Kelly Ann Jacobson, Oliver Gray, Eileen McGervey, Millie Kahn, and many, many others. To Cook Club, the best book club that never agreed on a book.

To my family and my in-laws: you've shown me how to love every single part of creating, and caring for, my own family. To Casey especially, forever in our hearts.

And finally, of course, to Jack and our son. Thank you for sharing joy in what we didn't expect.

About the Contributors

Becky Charniak received her bachelor's degree in political science with a minor in writing from the Johns Hopkins University, and her master's degree in political theory from Northwestern University. She has served on the UMass Memorial NICU Parent and Family Advisory Council. She lives in Massachusetts with her husband and two daughters.

Sara Cohen worked in a level-4 NICU in Philadelphia for fourteen years before obtaining her master's degree in nursing education and becoming a nurse educator. She now helps the hospital staff learn and perfect procedures in their clinical environment, from total body cooling in the NICU to rapid transfusions in the emergency department, and anything in between. She is also a volunteer peer support parent for Parent to Parent PA, a program linking parents of children with various medical conditions to peer supporters who have personal or professional experience with the same conditions.

Tyrese Coleman's debut collection of stories and essays, *How to Sit,* was nominated for a 2019 PEN Open Book Award, and her second book, *Spectacle,* will be published by One World. Her articles and essays have appeared in BuzzFeed, *Brain, Child* magazine, *Black Warrior Review, The Kenyon Review,* LitHub, *Washingtonian,* The Rumpus, Rewire News, Electric Literature, and *Atticus Review,* and she is the reviews editor for *SmokeLong Quarterly.* Her work was a notable in *Best American Essays 2018* and nominated for a Pushcart Prize. She received her bachelor's degree in English language and literature from the University of Maryland in College Park, her J.D. from the University of Baltimore, and her master's degree in writing from the Johns Hopkins University.

Sarah DiGregorio is the author of *Early: An Intimate History of Premature Birth and What It Teaches Us About Being Human*, published by Harper in 2020, and the forthcoming *Taking Care: An Essential History of the Nurse*. Before becoming a freelance journalist, she was a staff writer at the *Village Voice* and an editor at *Food & Wine* and BuzzFeed.

Ashley Franklin is the author of *Not Quite Snow White* (2019), "Creative Fixes" from the anthology *Once Upon an Eid* (2020), and *Better Together, Cinderella* (2021). She received her master's degree in English literature from the University of Delaware and is now an adjunct college instructor and proud mom. She currently resides in Arkansas with her family.

Jonathan Freeman-Coppadge is the fiction editor at *Oyster River Pages* and a high school English teacher. His latest work appears in *Embark Literary Journal*, *Italian Americana*, and *Rainbow in the Word: LGBTQ Christians' Biblical Memoirs* (Wipf and Stock, 2017). He lives with his husband and their son in Maryland.

Manuel Hernandez is a twenty-three-year-old screenwriter and filmmaker who just graduated from college, to the unending pride of his parents.

Pramila Jayapal represents Washington state's Seventh District in the U.S. House of Representatives and serves as the cochair of the Congressional Progressive Caucus. Jayapal came to the United States by herself at the age of sixteen to attend college at Georgetown University, and she later received her master's in business administration from Northwestern University. Prior to serving in elected office, she spent twenty years working internationally and domestically in global public health and development. She is the author of *Pilgrimage to India: A Woman Revisits Her Homeland* and *Use the Power You Have: A Brown Woman's Guide to Politics and Political Change*.

Suzanne Kamata is the author or editor of ten published books, including the novel *Losing Kei*; the anthologies *Love You to Pieces: Creative Writers on Raising a Child with Special Needs* and *Call Me Okaasan: Adventures in Multicultural Mothering*; and the memoir *Squeaky Wheels: Travels with My Daughter by Train, Plane, Metro, Tuk-tuk and Wheelchair* (Wyatt-Mackenzie Publishing, 2019). Her essays have appeared in *Real Simple, Brain, Child, Hippocampus*, and *One Big Happy Family* (Riverhead, 2009).

Dan Koboldt has three jobs. As a genetics researcher, he has coauthored more than eighty publications in *Nature, Science, The New England Journal of Medicine*, and other scientific journals. As a science fiction and fantasy writer, he's the author of the *Gateways to Alissia* series with Harper Voyager (2016–2018) and the editor of *Putting the Science in Fiction* (Writers Digest, 2018). As a husband and father, he's read countless children's books out loud and told more bedtime stories than he can possibly remember.

Janine Kovac is a former professional ballet dancer and software engineer. Her memoir, *SPINNING: Choreography for Coming Home*, was a 2019 winner for the National Indie Excellence Awards and a semifinalist for *Publishers Weekly*'s BookLife Prize. She is a recipient of the Elizabeth George Foundation Fellowship, and her thesis "A Cognitive Linguistic Analysis of Parenting" received the Robert J. Glushko Award for Distinguished Research in Cognitive Science from the University of California Berkeley. Her current project is a collection of essays about a family of five that dances in *The Nutcracker*. She lives with her family in Oakland, California.

Kelsey Osgood is the author of the 2013 book *How to Disappear Completely*, which was chosen for the Barnes and Noble Discover Great New Writers program. As a journalist, she has contributed to *Harper's, The New Yorker*, Jezebel, *Time*, and *New York*, among other outlets. She was a consultant to David Kessler, former head of the U.S. Food and Drug Administration, on his book *Capture: Unraveling the Mystery of Mental Suffering.*

Maria Ramos-Chertok is the founder and facilitator of The Butterfly Series, an online writing workshop supporting women's creativity and ability to access their inner wisdom. As an executive coach, she supports nonprofit leaders working for social justice, and since 2008 she has been part of the training team of Rockwood Leadership Institute. A graduate of the University of Pennsylvania School of Law, her legal work is focused on sexual harassment prevention. She is currently working on her next book, *Woman Being: Incantations on Freedom.*

Shawn Spruce is a Native American economic and community development consultant. A member of the Laguna Pueblo in west central New Mexico, he currently resides with his family in Asheville, North Carolina.

Anne Thériault is a Toronto-based writer whose bylines can be found all over the internet, including at *The Guardian*, the *London Review of Books*, and Longreads. She truly believes that your favorite Tudor wife says more about you than your astrological sign. She is currently raising one child and three unruly cats.

Megan Walker is the author of *A Beautiful Love* and *Lakeshire Park*. Walker graduated from Brigham Young University with a degree in early childhood education. She currently resides in St. Louis, Missouri, with her husband and their children.

Melody Schreiber has reported from nearly every continent, covering everything from the effects of climate change on mental health in the Arctic to the changing tides of livelihoods in the Chesapeake Bay. She is the D.C. correspondent for ArcticToday, and her work has also been published by *The Washington Post, The Guardian, Wired, The Atlantic, Pacific Standard, USA Today, Outside, The New Republic*, NPR, and elsewhere. She was awarded journalism fellowships from the International Women's Media Foundation (IWMF) in 2019 and the GroundTruth Project in 2015–2016. Schreiber received her bachelor's degree in English and linguistics from Georgetown University, and her master's degree in writing from the Johns Hopkins University.